THE
Everyday Ayurveda
Cookbook

Also by Kate O'Donnell

Everyday Ayurveda Cooking for a Calm,
Clear Mind: 100 Simple Sattvic Recipes

Everyday Ayurveda for Women's Health: Traditional
Wisdom, Recipes, and Remedies for Optimal Wellness,
Hormone Balance, and Living Radiantly

The Everyday Ayurveda Guide to Self-Care: Rhythms,
Routines, and Home Remedies for Natural Healing

THE
Everyday Ayurveda
Cookbook

A Seasonal Guide to Eating and Living Well

TENTH ANNIVERSARY EDITION

KATE O'DONNELL

with CARA BROSTROM

Foreword by AMADEA MORNINGSTAR

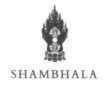

SHAMBHALA

Shambhala Publications, Inc.
2129 13th Street
Boulder, Colorado 80302
www.shambhala.com

Cover art: Cara Brostrom
Cover design: Kate E. White
Interior design: Allison Meierding

9 8 7 6 5 4 3 2 1
Second Edition

Printed in China

Shambhala Publications makes every effort to print on acid-free, recycled paper.
Shambhala Publications is distributed worldwide by Penguin Random House, Inc., and its subsidiaries.

Library of Congress Cataloging-in-Publication Data
Names: O'Donnell, Kate (Ayurvedic practitioner) author. | Brostrom, Cara, photographer. | Morningstar, Amadea, 1952– writer of foreword.
Title: The everyday Ayurveda cookbook: a seasonal guide to eating and living well / Kate O'Donnell; photography by Cara Brostrom; foreword by Amadea Morningstar.
Description: Second edition. | Boulder, Colorado: Shambhala, 2025. | Includes bibliographical references and index.
Identifiers: LCCN 2024009180 | ISBN 9781645473411 (trade paperback)
Subjects: LCSH: Vegetarianism. | Vegetarian cooking. | Seasonal cooking. | Medicine, Ayurvedic. | LCGFT: Cookbooks.
Classification: LCC RM236 .O34 2025 | DDC 613.2/62—dc23/eng/20240411
LC record available at https://lccn.loc.gov/2024009180

THIS BOOK IS DEDICATED TO THE AYUR VIDYA,
THE SPIRIT OF AYURVEDA.

Contents

Foreword

When Kate O'Donnell wrote *The Everyday Ayurveda Cookbook* ten years ago, it was a game changer. It was (and is!) very well organized and beautiful, with a great presentation of Ayurveda principles. The recipes can be readily adapted to other cultures and conditions, a real plus in these times and for the spread of Ayurveda. Knowledge about Ayurveda healing has expanded outward tremendously from South Asia over the last forty years. So many people have worked together to make this possible.

When I first began working on *The Ayurvedic Cookbook* in the late eighties with my coauthor, Urmila Desai, there were no resource books in English about Ayurveda nutrition. We wanted the information to be accurate and the recipes to be flavorful and easy to digest. It was important to us that the healing properties of foods be clearly described and that we not steer anyone astray! Work on this book began prior to the Internet. I lived in a rural area in a mountain canyon in northern New Mexico with a "party line" (shared phone with an operator). From Kripalu in Massachusetts, my coauthor *Mataji* (Urmila Desai) would mail me sheets of paper with various ingredients for her recipes taped to them. We would discuss the project and the dynamics of the foods and dishes with the phone operator listening in on us. It was a different time.

When *The Everyday Ayurveda Cookbook* was published, it inspired me as an experienced Ayurveda cook to think creatively. As an educator, it made me wonder how I could make my own recipes and blog simpler. It upped the ante. When teaching or writing about Ayurveda, I'd ask, *How can I make this visually appealing as well as informative?* I thank Kate and Cara for this uplift.

The Everyday Ayurveda Cookbook is beautifully simple and tasty, and easy to use. It is well-suited to meet the needs of these coming years of change. In working with simplicity, we need to have the wisdom to see what is essential and what is extraneous. Kate and Cara have done this in outstanding ways, and this cookbook continues to encourage us to be wise and simple.

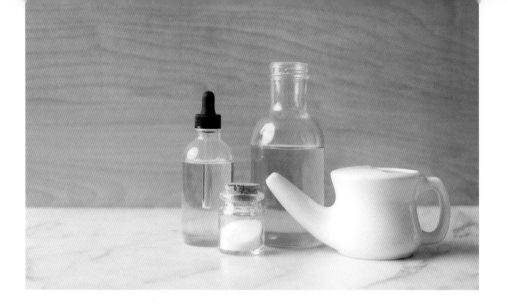

In my forty years of this work, I've seen that there are many ways to engage with Ayurveda. As Kate says, "Reading about Ayurveda may help you understand its principles, but it is not until you start experimenting with its diet and lifestyle recommendations that you will begin to see improvements in your health." I wholeheartedly agree. May these efforts be of benefit.

With glad blessings to these my Ayurveda sisters and you, dear reader,

Amadea Morningstar, MA, RPE, RYT
author of *The Ayurvedic Cookbook* and
Easy Healing Drinks from the Wisdom of Ayurveda

Author's Note on the Tenth Anniversary Edition

Amadea Morningstar's work in Ayurveda cooking and nutrition was seminal for me. I have memories of sitting in bed, pouring over her paperback cookbooks, full of information about how Ayurveda uses food as medicine, along with simple and nourishing recipes.

Ten years after the publication of *The Everyday Ayurveda Cookbook*, I can now envision so many of you, readers, holding this book as I did Amadea's. I have met thousands of you at workshops and book signings, and I have seen your dog-eared, sticky-noted, food-spattered copies. You tell me it's your Ayurveda "bible," so much more than a cookbook, a resource that has healed, inspired, and supported you and your families. It is so affirming to hear that the resource Cara and I set out to create has truly changed you.

Upon hearing a client say for the hundredth time, "I have an Ayurveda cookbook, but I don't use it because I don't know my dosha," I had thrown up my hands and said to Cara, "We need a new cookbook!" The next day, an acquiring editor from Shambhala, also a former client, reached out to ask, "Have you thought about doing a cookbook?" Well, if that wasn't a sign....

After an unprecedented two-year hustle, *The Everyday Ayurveda Cookbook* emerged at the crest of a breaking wave of new publications and media exposure for the ancient science of Ayurveda. My work has been featured on national news, in fashion magazines, and at major retail outlets. Recently, I've seen bookstores with Ayurveda sections on the shelves and Ayurveda listed in annual top-ten wellness trends, which is thrilling.

As we celebrate ten years together—of healing, transforming, and nourishing ourselves and our loved ones—I'd like to deeply thank you, readers, for taking this book into your home and getting down to business in the kitchen with me. We have come so far together, and yet a lifetime

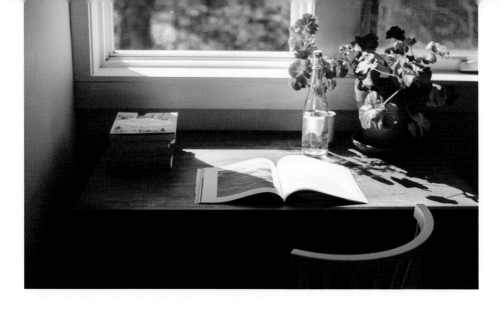

of purposeful work still remains to continue to transform daily fare into healing alchemy. Stick with me, readers. Let's walk this path, doing a little bit every day to improve our physical, mental, and spiritual health, and bring positivity to the space around us.

Kate O'Donnell
2024

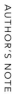

Reader's Note

Food has always been a friend. I have been playing with food since, as Mom tells me, I made mud pies on the front steps of our house. By an auspicious twist of fate, I came of age in the kitchens of India. I first visited the subcontinent in college, when I was beginning to learn how to cook for myself. Hanging around in village kitchens and trying my hand at rolling chapati and frying up *dosa* is how I learned—and I still don't know how to cook a good mac and cheese. But I don't eat much cheese or pasta. Because it feels good to eat these things and supports my early morning yoga practice, my staples are dal, basmati rice, and *kichari*. This book will teach you how to make all these things and more.

I never thought too much about digestion, but after a few years of the traveling lifestyle, it seemed like most foods didn't make me feel well, and I began to notice the connection between what I ate and my state of being. When my digestion became critical in India during one trip, I found an Ayurvedic doctor who taught me about how the system uses foods for healing. Once he wrote down the name of a recommended vegetable in the local language, and I brought the piece of paper to the vegetable vendor. He pointed to a white squash the size of a ceiling fan. He sawed off a wedge and wrapped it in newspaper, and I took it home to my kitchen. Here began my hobby of creating recipes to showcase medicinal foods, finding context for the different grains, pulses, fruits, and vegetables recommended in the Ayurvedic diet. My cooking with unfamiliar items found in the street markets of India, and with local foods from the farmers' markets at home, makes up the years of culinary research behind these recipes.

Fast-forward fifteen years. I live in the city. I am a full-time yoga teacher and Ayurvedic practitioner. The diet and lifestyle I introduce in this book have greatly supported me in sustaining a life of service in an urban environment and in balancing a spiritual path with the duties of daily life. I take good care of myself so I can show up consistently to support communities that experience the depth and gifts of yoga and Ayurveda amid a modern-paced life. The Ayurvedic principle of eating digestible foods in a calm environment remains, for me, the key to staying healthy and vibrant.

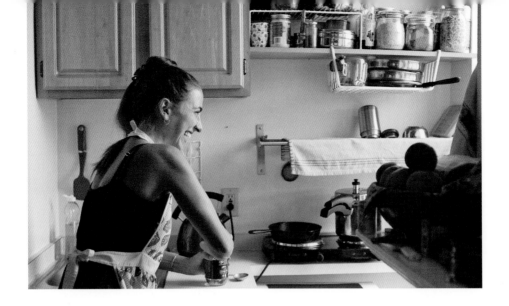

This is real life; I get busy, and I get hungry. Out of necessity I have birthed hybridized versions of the cookery of India in my tiny apartment kitchens. *The Everyday Ayurveda Cookbook* uses fresh, seasonal ingredients to enable you to create, in the middle of a busy day, authentic, healing meals.

Photographer Cara Brostrom began making some of my recipes at home to get her body in balance. Her experience of Ayurveda was so beneficial, she offered her talents to help me get the word out (and to get organized). Her countless hours of cooking and editing the recipes keep them stylish and delicious, whereas in my own kitchen, quick and easy are at the top of the list. All of the photos in this book are of meals Cara and I made and then ate. She kept the Everyday Ayurveda component at the forefront and took pictures of real food made in real time, so you can truly expect your cooking to look like the pictures. Cara's own experiential understanding of Ayurveda translates into the beauty and simplicity you see in this book.

I invite you to step into my urban-village kitchen and learn about Ayurvedic cookery by doing it, like I did. I've seen it help a lot of people, a lot of people have helped me along the way, and now it's your turn to roll up the sleeves and fry some dosa. This book offers not only recipes, seasonal food guides, and shopping lists but also simple, strategic guidelines to get you started practicing Ayurvedic cooking and lifestyle routines right away. I want these ancient principles for health and happiness to slip into your life seamlessly. It's simple, and it's possible. Let's do it together, every day.

Kate O'Donnell
Boston, MA
2014

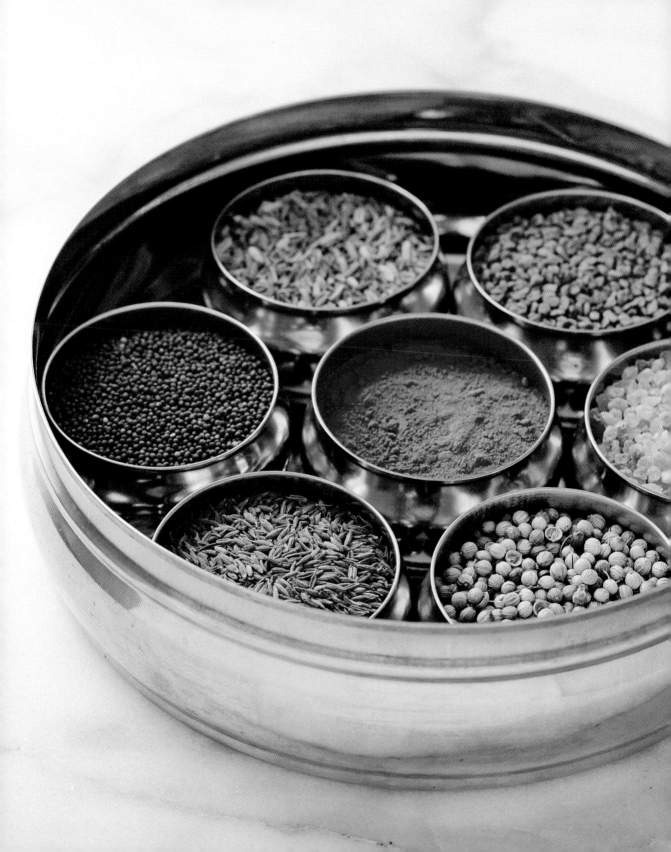

Introduction

ABOUT *THE EVERYDAY AYURVEDA COOKBOOK*

Here's what this book is meant to do: get you in the kitchen. Not for big projects, but for simple preparations, most days. Maybe even every day. You may or may not fall in love with cooking, but it's important to know that preparing food for yourself is a key element of wellness. This book will keep it simple, practical, and functional. The goal is not to create fancy or perfect meals but to be satisfied by your food. Some days this may mean having a treat; other days it may mean keeping your food really basic to serve as fuel for your day. The food program in this book provides plenty of variety, but it is based on simplicity.

Ayurveda is the indigenous health science of India, a way of understanding balance and imbalance in the body so that we can avoid the progression of disease by addressing the causes early on. The inspiration behind *The Everyday Ayurveda Cookbook* is to demystify this ancient science, which truly has something in it to help everyone. A huge part of staying healthy, in the Ayurveda view, lies in proper digestion and nutrition. The foods we eat become the tissues of the body, and the attitudes we bring to the table contribute to the body's ability to digest and integrate food nicely. Being aware of what the body needs as we choose our foods and wishing the body well as we prepare them go a long way toward helping us feeling good.

This book is for you if you are:
- Looking for concrete ways to improve your diet and lifestyle
- New to Ayurveda or to cooking in general
- Feeling tired or anxious or experiencing poor digestion
- Interested in applying a traditional, holistic healing system to your life

The following chapters greatly simplify what is a complete, sophisticated, tried-and-true medical science by focusing on a few general points that we all can apply to set the stage for healthy living. Ayurveda is a symphony of experiential knowledge, and you are getting a hit single here, one that may inspire you to buy the album someday. But even if you don't, this book can change your life.

The recipes here also offer a simplified approach to the art of cooking, specifically Ayurvedic cooking, in which all food can be medicine. I've pared down any traditional dishes with long lists of ingredients or too many stages of preparation, so that you can make the recipes without a lot of fuss. This simplicity will empower you to enjoy eating something you've made for yourself, every day. It is possible.

WHAT YOU WILL FIND IN THIS BOOK:
- An introduction to Ayurveda and how this diet and lifestyle work, though you don't need to read it (let alone memorize it) to use this book to your advantage.
- Methods for making simple breakfasts, lunches, and suppers that can be adapted by changing key ingredients as the seasons change.
- Daily self-care routines for each season and suggestions of what time of day to practice them.
- Shopping lists for each season, which will set you up to make all of the staple recipes in each seasonal chapter.
- Travel tips, family tips, and take-it-to-work tips for eating well and staying on center during your regular routine.
- Tried-and-true practices for improving the function of the digestive organs (and feeling good after you eat).
- A walk-through of safe spring and fall cleansing practices.

PRAKRITI, YOUR TRUE NATURE

Ayurveda is known for its individualized approach: each person is seen as a unique system with unique needs and tendencies. *Prakriti* means "nature." This word is used to encompass all primordial matter, what you might call Mother Nature, and *prakriti* refers to one's individual, true nature. *You are made up of a unique combination of nature's elements, and the qualities of these elements in your body make you who, and how, you are!* Understanding what elements are prevalent in your body is intuitive, and the recipes in this book will help you feel how the elements manifest in you. Take some time to let the practices in this book settle in, and if you want to know more, an Ayurvedic practitioner can help you further understand how certain elements may have tendencies to get out of balance in your body and teach you how to manage these specific tendencies through diet and lifestyle.

WHAT YOU WON'T FIND IN THIS BOOK:

- Complicated recipes that require you to buy expensive ingredients
- Recipes that contain white sugar or refined flours
- Heavy use of nightshade vegetables (tomatoes, eggplants, bell peppers, white potatoes), a family of vegetables containing trace amounts of toxins, which can build up and promote inflammation in some bodies
- Reliance on garlic and raw onion for seasoning, as both are heating foods and encourage an excitable mind
- Information on personal constitutions and disease diagnosis. For this, you'll need to consult other resources or an Ayurvedic practitioner (see "Resources," page 320).

Roots of the Recipes

TRADITIONAL

Many of the recipes in this book are inspired by cookery I learned in India, either in households or at Ayurveda centers and clinics. The Ayurvedic sensibility is ingrained in the cookery of India, though one has to go into private homes to find it. Most of the food served in restaurants, both in India and in Indian restaurants abroad, does not represent healthy eating. Modern media is changing sensibilities about diet in India, as it does in Western countries. Propaganda paid for by manufacturers distributes new ideas regarding what is "good for you" on a regular basis. Problems of obesity and diabetes are accompanying changes in the economy of modern India. People in the home country of Ayurveda, as well as in the Western world, are looking to this ancient system of well-being for unbiased recommendations based on thousands of years of discovering what works.

REGIONAL

Some of the indigenous ingredients mentioned by classic Ayurvedic texts are unavailable outside of India. To mirror the medicinal qualities by using what is available, I've modified the recipes in this book with local foods, finding what worked by trial and error. In some cases, a standby recipe with its roots in New England culture, such as Kate's Apple Crisp or Yam and Oat Muffins, represents my intuitive knowledge of the culinary ancestry in New England. No doubt, wherever you are living, or whatever your family may have taught you, a cookery to support the climate and lifestyle of a people is present. Any regional diet will favor cooking with foods indigenous to the area. I encourage you to experiment with making *Everyday Ayurveda* recipes with your local produce. With a little practice, you can also begin to modify your family recipes to integrate Ayurvedic principles.

HEALTH NUT

An Ayurveda cookbook with a recipe for Tofu Tacos with Greens? In the mission to help you feel at home in this cookbook, I have included some Western-style meals and modern ingredients, like chia seeds. One is not required to eat Indian food all the time to be Ayurvedically sound, and with the creativity of melting-pot cultures, many culinary gems have emerged, some of them quite convenient to make and a shame to leave out of an Everyday cookbook. I have modified the recipes to respect Ayurvedic digestive recommendations, such as food combining, cooking methods, and the beneficial use of digestive spices.

Behind *The Everyday Ayurveda Cookbook* recipes stand twenty years I've spent working in health food stores and cafes, modifying recipes to include every health food product under the sun. Recipes including Western health foods ingredients, such as sea vegetables, tacos made with tofu, and sunflower seed butter, do not appear in traditional Ayurvedic cooking, but they are staples in my own kitchen and adhere to Ayurvedic principles.

For some people, developing a taste for Indian flavors will take some time, especially the sweets. In truth, Indian desserts are a tough sell for the Western palate. Try the Coconut Rice Pudding (known in India as *kheer*) and the Saffron Lassi. But when you are looking for a familiar comfort treat, you may rely on my Ayurveda-inspired versions of well-known favorites, such as Kate's Apple Crisp and Almond Ginger Macaroons. Hey, I'm here for you, keeping you happy and healthy with special recipes for treats, without the refined flours and sugars Ayurveda warns against.

The Everyday Ayurveda Cookbook has two parts: part one is the theory, and part two is the practice. Feel free to dive into the practice chapters (get cooking!) and poke around in part one, as your interest in Ayurveda expands.

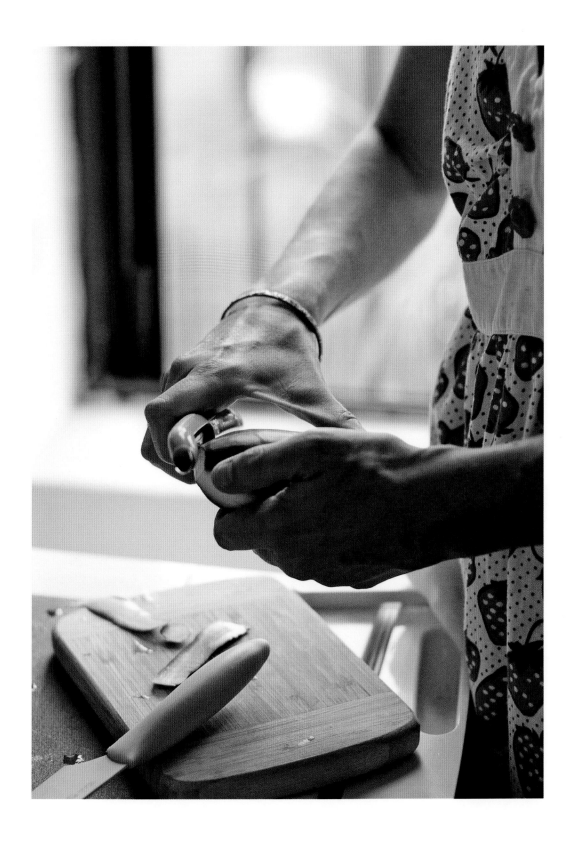

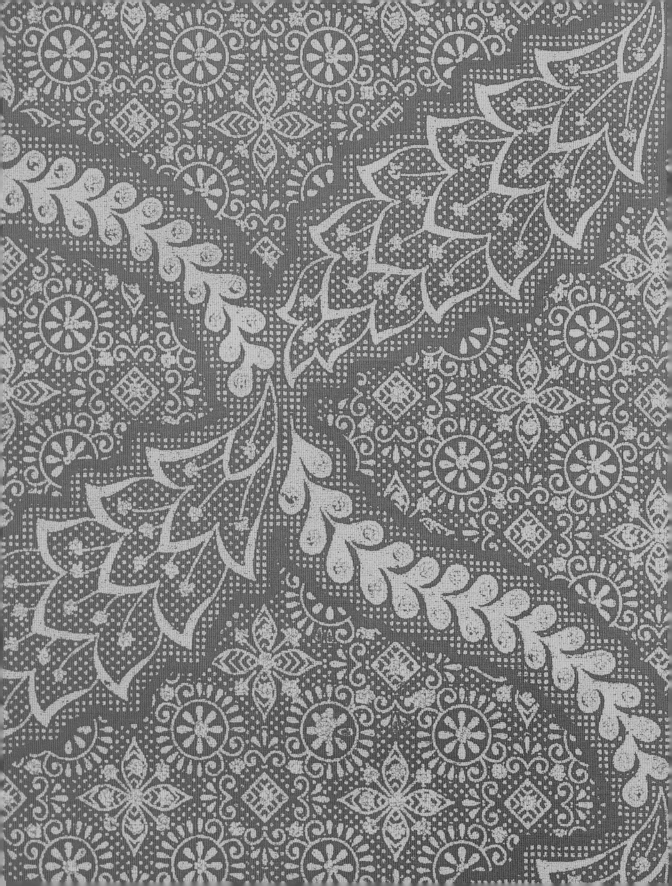

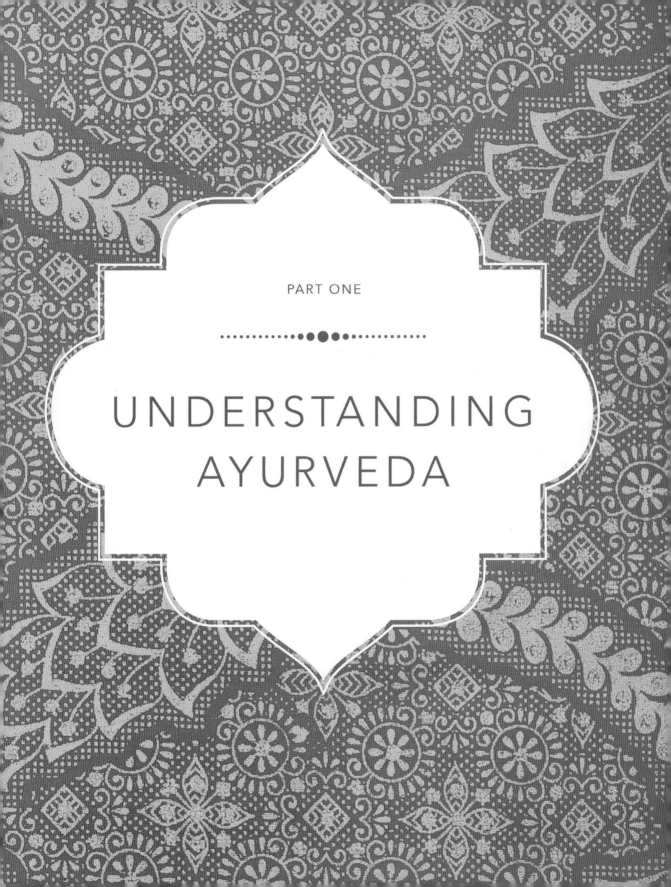

PART ONE

· · · · · · · · · • ● • · · · · · · · · ·

UNDERSTANDING AYURVEDA

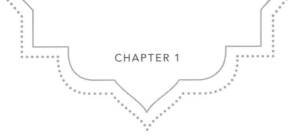

CHAPTER 1

Ayurveda Basics
You Want to Know

One of the best things about Ayurveda is how simple it is … and one of the funniest things about simplicity is how complicated we can make it! The following introduction to Ayurveda is for those who are interested and for those who are more likely to integrate changes in their diets and lifestyles if they have some understanding of how a suggestion proves beneficial.

References to classic Ayurvedic texts are also included, to ensure we don't forget this information about healthy living comes from an extremely reliable source: thousands of years of human trial and error.

You don't even have to read this chapter to benefit from this book. Maybe you are holding *The Everyday Ayurveda Cookbook* because you know your eating habits could use some improvement. That sounds great. The seasonal chapters in part two provide enough basic information to keep you eating foods that will maintain balance throughout the year's changing seasons, without your having to think too hard about it. An intuitive understanding of the science of Ayurveda is sure to follow. The lifestyle grows with experience, so start with the cooking.

But if you do want to read about the tools before you try them, let us begin a journey into Ayurveda.

What Is Ayurveda?

Pronounced "EYE-yer-VAY-da," *Ayurveda* can be loosely translated as "the science of life." The classic texts, however, describe *Ayur*, or "life," as being made up of four parts: the physical body, the mind, the soul, and the senses (sight, hearing, touch, smell, and taste). Contrary to the Western model, which focuses on the physical body, and sometimes on the mind these days, Ayurveda has always taken into account the health of these four aspects of life.

Ayurveda, the health system of India, employs diet, biorhythms, herbal medicine, psychology, wholesome lifestyle, surgery, and therapeutic bodywork to address the root causes of disease. The science describes the disease process from early symptoms to fatality, and it includes prevention and treatments for ailments of eight therapeutic branches: internal medicine; surgery; gynecology/obstetrics/pediatrics; two varieties of geriatrics, rejuvenation of the body and rejuvenation of the sexual energy; psychology; toxicology; and disorders of the eyes, ears, nose, and mouth.

Ayurvedic hospitals and clinics abound in India. Western medicine is often used in conjunction with the traditional medicine, especially in cases of critical ailments. While Western medicine excels at resolving acute situations, Ayurveda excels as a preventive medicine, seeking to halt the progression from imbalance to disease by addressing the underlying causes early on. Used alongside Western medicine, Ayurveda can support digestion, the immune system, and the patient's state of mind during treatment.

Where Does It Come From?

Ayurveda may be the oldest continually practiced health system in the world. The knowledge, in its current state, is believed to be anywhere from two to five thousand years old, depending on whom you talk to. The earliest information on Ayurveda is contained in the *Rig-Veda*, one of four bodies of ancient scripture, orally transmitted in lyrical phrases called *sutras* (threads). The Vedas are believed to originate from the rishis, sages in deep states of meditation. The Vedas contain information on music, mantras, ritual worship, Ayurveda, and yoga.

Of the several classical Sanskrit texts (Sanskrit is the language of ancient India) that make up the body of Ayurvedic science, three are

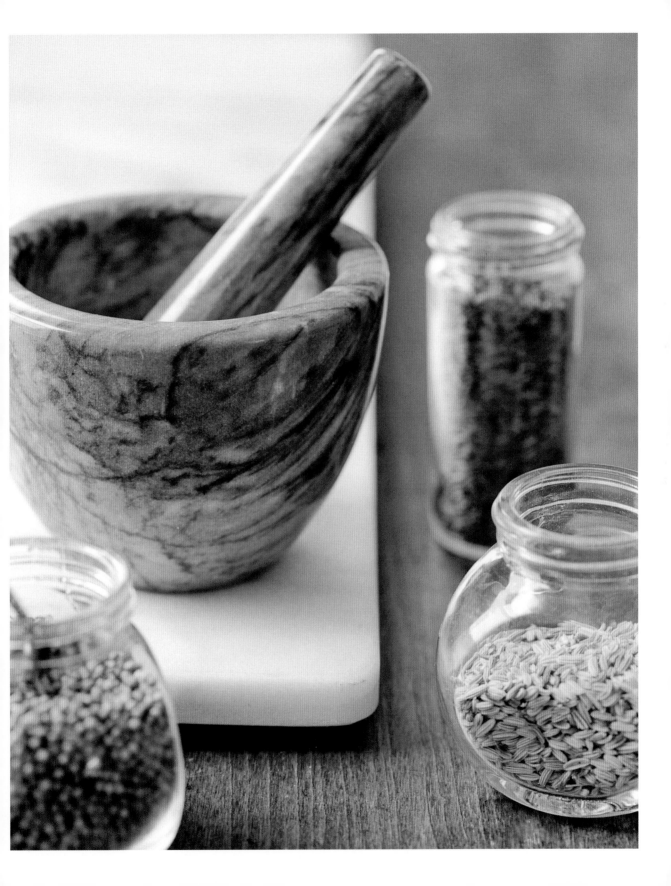

most important: the Charaka Samhita, the Sushruta Samhita, and the Ashtanga Hridayam (a compilation of Charaka and Sushruta). All have been translated into English, and this book will occasionally reference the Ashtanga Hridayam.

How Does It Work?

Ayurveda recognizes that the human being is a microcosm (a small part; a reflection) of the macrocosm (the big picture; the universe). The human body is made up of the same elements that make up everything else around us, and we are moved by the same energies or forces that move the oceans, the winds, the stars, and the planets.

This world operates in rhythm—for example, the cycles of the sun, moon, tides, and seasons—and so do we. The introduction of artificial light, global food transportation, and a schedule so busy that we don't notice nature's rhythms makes it easy to get out of sync.

If a person acts as if he or she is separate from the rhythms of the macrocosm, marching to his or her own drummer (by eating tropical fruits in winter, for example, or foods primarily from bags and boxes; staying up all night; and/or breathing recycled air), the organism will get wacky. If the movements of our world are a river we are floating in, why swim upstream? You start to feel tired, don't digest your food well, and, over time, end up "out of order."

What's Food Got to Do with It?

Digestion is of paramount importance in Ayurveda. The complete digestion, absorption, and assimilation of food nutrients make up the building blocks of the body, called *ahara rasa*, the juice of the food. When the food is chewed and swallowed, it mixes with water, enzymes, and acids. The resulting product—food matter ready to be assimilated—is the "juice." To assimilate nature's bounty into the body connects the microcosm to the macrocosm. Good digestion results not only in a glowing, healthy body but in a glowing consciousness as well. If you are just beginning to understand Ayurveda, it may be easier to become aware of what you are eating and how it makes you feel than it is to realize whether you are "connected." The feelings of connection and wholeness are fostered by a good diet and a good gut, and isn't that what everybody wants?

What's It Got to Do with Yoga?

Yoga and Ayurveda stem from the same philosophical roots and evolved at around the same time in history. They also share the same goal: to create a union between microcosm and macrocosm. The philosophy of yoga provides a pathway for navigating the mind/body organism toward an understanding of itself as being unified with the universe. The science of Ayurveda focuses primarily on maintaining the physical body, but the link between consciousness and health is clear. Yoga, popular these days for its physical benefits, has traditionally focused more on accessing the mental and energy bodies. Yoga movements and breathing techniques may be employed by Ayurveda to stimulate an organ or system of organs or to ease stress. The further one journeys down the limb of Ayurveda that specializes in psychology, the more one is likely to run into the philosophical system of yoga.

NOTE: This book is for beginners to the Ayurvedic lifestyle and diet, who want to home in on general foods and practices for the annual cycle. The subject of yoga and Ayurveda could fill an entire book on its own and so is not covered here.

How Does Ayurveda View the Body?

In Ayurveda, human anatomy starts with the five elements: space (also called "ether"), air, fire, water, and earth. The elements create three compounds that govern specific functions and energies in the body, namely: movement, transformation, and cohesion (holding things together). When these compounds, known as *doshas*, are in balance and working harmoniously, the individual will enjoy smooth moving processes (digestion, circulation, etc.), clear senses, proper elimination of wastes, and happiness (satisfaction, fulfillment).

Each of these five elemental compounds manifests as certain felt qualities in the body that one can recognize simply by paying attention to bodily sensations. For example, air and space are cold and light, fire is hot and sharp, and earth and water are heavy and moist. Too much or too little of a grouping of qualities brings on imbalance in the body. A prevalence of dry and light qualities, for instance, will result in dry skin. *Ayurveda manages imbalance by introducing opposite qualities and reducing like qualities.* In the case of dry skin, introducing moist, heavy foods and reducing dry and light foods will alleviate the symptom.

Remember: this book deliberately keeps things simple, but we are talking about a profound system. Know that classical Ayurveda describes all of the channels that transport substances and information throughout the body, as well as the progression of disease in six stages. It has well-defined preventive applications and treatments for disease at each stage of its progression. Although Ayurveda does provide very useful home remedies, this is not folklore but a medical science.

Read on to learn about keeping your system of elements, doshas, and qualities in balance.

Pancha Mahabhutas, The Five Elements

Ayurveda views the human body, as well as all forms in our universe, as being made up of differing combinations of the five elements:

- Space
- Air
- Fire
- Water
- Earth

For example, a carrot contains space, gases, the heat of the sun, and water, and its structure—hard, orange colored, and fibrous—is made of earth. A human body, like everything in the cosmos, comprises all five elements working together. Use your own body as a frame of reference for understanding the five elements.

Space. Every body has lots of space in it—usually filled with something like food, acid, fluid, and/or waste products.
- The large intestine, and indeed the entire digestive channel from the mouth to the anus, is a long, cavernous space! Without that space there, where would we put food?
- The ear, that delicate organ that sounds bounce around inside of.
- The bones are porous, hard tissue with hollow interiors, which are filled with marrow.
- The skin, our largest organ, is exposed to the qualities of space all of the time.

Air. Anywhere there is movement, there is air. Space is passive, while air moves around. And anywhere there is space, air will move. You can feel air on your skin when a breeze blows and see it moving the clouds across the sky.

- Respiration is the movement of air in and out of the nose or mouth.
- Passing gas and belching are caused by movements of air out of the intestine and stomach, respectively. If you eat excitedly, excess air is likely to get in your mouth, and you will be gassier. Bubbly drinks make you burp because you are ingesting air with your liquid.
- The sound of cracking joints is made by air moving out from the spaces between the bones.

Fire. On earth, anywhere there is heat, fire is there: a hot spring, a lightning bolt, a forest blaze. Fire of the sun warms the earth, as it does a human body. The core of the earth is fire, just as is the human core, the stomach and small intestine. Anywhere there is heat in the body, it comes from fire.

- The stomach and small intestine are fire centers: the acids and enzymes they produce are hot.
- The blood is characterized by fire, especially if you are "hot-blooded."
- The metabolism and some hormones are hot. (Think puberty or pregnancy.)
- The function of the eye requires fire. Consider how your eyes can get hot, red, and dry if you spend too much time on the computer or in front of the TV.

Water. Water is all over the planet, in rivers, oceans, the cells of plants, and humans. As you probably know, some 80 percent of the body is made up of water, and you are filled with liquids.

- All of the mucous membranes, which cover the digestive tract, the eyes, and the sinuses, rely on water.
- The lymphatic fluid flowing through your body has a base of water.
- Blood in your circulatory system contains water.
- Digestive juices require water.
- Synovial fluid lubricating the joints is the water element keeping you juicy.
- Saliva is water flowing into the mouth for the first stage of digestion.

Earth. In nature, earth is anything solid—soil, rocks, trees, and the flesh of animals. This is the solid structure of the body and the easiest element, conceptually, to wrap your head around: it's all the meaty stuff.

- Adipose tissue (aka fat) is extra earth element being stored.
- Muscle fiber is the earth element holding your skeleton in place.
- The stable part of your bones (not the space inside), which makes up the structure of your skeleton, is composed of the earth element.

It's important to remember that the same five elements are moving around in all of us and in everything. We are all made of the same stuff, which is why Ayurveda views the human organism as a microcosm of the whole universe. When we eat a carrot and transform it by absorbing and assimilating its elements into our tissues, the body takes those elements of the carrot and incorporates them into its own structure, thus linking our bodies to the world outside.

REMEMBER: digestion is the most important aspect of health. If we are digesting soundly, we will feel connected to the greater whole. If the body has a hard time breaking down the carrot and making something out of it, we will feel separate, unsatisfied, tired, and eventually pretty crappy.

The Three Doshas: Functional Friends

Most people who have heard of Ayurveda have heard of the doshas. *Dosha* literally means "that which is at fault."[1] But doshas aren't a problem until imbalance has been hanging around in the body awhile. These energies do good or ill, depending on whether they are in a relative state of balance. That's why it is more important to understand how to maintain balance than it is to dwell on doshas as the bad guys.

There are three doshas, known as *vata, pitta,* and *kapha.* These are the compounds that naturally arise when the five elements come together in certain combinations to make up a human organism. Each performs a specific function in the body and manifests as a recognizable grouping of qualities.

VATA (*VA-tah*) is the energy of movement.

PITTA (*PITT-ah*) is the energy of transformation.

KAPHA (*CUP-hah*) is the energy of structure and lubrication together; cohesion (think glue).

VATA

Where there is space, air begins to move, and the compound qualities of space and air manifest as *cold, light, dry, rough, mobile, erratic,* and *clear.* Space and air have no heat, moisture, or heaviness, right? These qualities are inherent in fire, water, and earth instead.

The qualities of space and air are naturally going to act a certain way and have certain effects on the body. Think of vata as the currents of the body. The body knows the food goes in the mouth, then down and out. It is vata that ushers it along. There is nothing problematic about the qualities of space and air or their function. However, if a body has accumulated too many of these qualities, certain aspects can get out of balance. For instance, the fall season is windy, dry, and cold, so the body gets this way after a little while (unless, of course, one is taking care to keep warm, eat warming, moist foods, and drink warm water). Too many vata qualities can result in signs of imbalance, such as gas and constipation, increasingly dry skin, and anxiety.

HEALTHY VATA ENSURES THAT THE BODY HAS

- Consistent elimination
- Free breathing
- Good circulation
- Keen senses

TOO MANY VATA QUALITIES MIGHT CAUSE

- Gas and constipation
- Constricted breathing
- Cold hands and feet
- Anxiety, feeling overwhelmed

PITTA

Where there is fire, there has to be water to keep it from burning everything up. The resulting compound is firewater, a *liquid, hot, sharp, penetrating, light, mobile, oily, smelly* grouping of qualities. (Think acid, bile.) When food gets chewed, pitta moves in to break it down, liquidize it, metabolize it, and transform it into tissues. Yee-haw! No problem with that, unless of course your internal environment gets too hot or too sharp, which can result in signs of imbalance such as acidy burps or reflux, diarrhea, skin rashes, or inflammation.

HEALTHY PITTA CREATES

- Good appetite and metabolism
- Steady hormones
- Sharp eyesight
- Comprehension
- Good complexion (rosy skin)

- Acid indigestion, reflux
- Dysmenorrhea
- Red, dry eyes; the need for glasses
- Tendency to overwork
- Acne, rosacea

KAPHA

Only when you add water to sand does it stick together so you can build a sand castle with it. The earth element requires water in this same way to get tissues to hold together. Kapha is like glue: *cool, liquid, slimy, heavy, slow, dull, dense,* and *stable.* This grouping of qualities provides density in the bones and fat, cohesion in the tissues and joints, and plenty of mucus so we don't dry out. Great! That is, unless the body becomes too heavy and too sticky, which can result in signs of imbalance such as loss of appetite, slow digestion, sinus troubles and allergies, or weight gain.

HEALTHY KAPHA PROVIDES

- Strong bodily tissues
- Hearty immune system
- Well-lubricated joints and mucous membranes

TOO MANY KAPHA QUALITIES MIGHT CAUSE

- Weight gain
- Water retention
- Sinus or lung congestion
- Lethargy and sadness

Every body should have a hearty dose of all of these qualities and thus healthy, well-functioning bodily processes. One person is more fiery and prone to an acid stomach, another is more spacey and prone to drying out—that's the truth of variation in nature. The body's constitution, or particular makeup of the five elements, is like DNA and comes mostly from one's parents. Understanding your constitution can help you understand which of the three compounds is likely to get out of balance in your body, so you can make choices in your diet and lifestyle that will keep your doshas in check.

It's easy to focus on dosha, that which is at fault. But categorizing oneself as a specific dosha ("I'm so vata") or identifying oneself with states of imbalance is not the aim of Ayurvedic wisdom. You may find it more helpful to understand and manage the general causes of imbalance first, and that's what *The Everyday Ayurveda Cookbook* will teach you how to do. Start with this and learn more about your individual constitution as your Ayurveda practices grow.

Nature's System of Checks and Balances: The Twenty Qualities

> There is no thing in this universe which is non-medicinal, which cannot be made use of for many purpose and by many modes.
> *Vagbhata, Ashtanga Hridayam, Sutrasthana 9.10*

Our world is made up of coexisting opposites. Like increases like, and opposites balance each other. The twenty qualities are how nature keeps a balance, and working with the qualities means you can help nature stay on course.

The qualities, or *gunas*, name the different attributes that are inherent in all substances. These pairs of opposing attributes identify the ways we feel and understand our world through comparison: it's hot or it's cool; it's sharp or it's smooth. Ayurveda has identified the ten pairs of opposites most useful as medicine. Moist and dry, heavy and light, cold and hot—all these pairings represent nature's system of checks and balances, present in all things, including the human body. When a quality or group of qualities is present in excess (the problem can also be depletion, but excess is more likely), imbalance can occur.

A pile of hot, sharp wasabi paste served without any cooling, smooth rice intuitively sounds a little off, doesn't it? Opposites balance each other. Ayurveda encourages balance by introducing qualities opposite to those promoting the imbalance, while reducing like qualities. For instance, one might enjoy a bit of spicy food to warm up in winter but avoid it in summer. All of the substances and experiences used as medicine (plants, meats, fruits, minerals, as well as activities) have an effect on the body, experienced as one or more of the twenty qualities. Spicy food makes you feel sweaty, and the effects of spicy food are heating and oily. The effects of lime are cool and light. See for yourself by drinking a Cardamom Limeade on a hot day (see page 195).

Once you start to think of your body's sensations or imbalances in terms of the qualities you are experiencing, you will be able to use food as medicine, introducing substances that have a balancing effect.

The qualities are divided into two important categories: *building* and *lightening*. The balance between these two energies in the body is central to maintaining an even keel and smooth bodily processes. Building qualities are anabolic. They build mass and nourish the tissues, encourage moisture, and strengthen, ground, and stabilize the body, mind, and nerves. Examples are comfort foods that make the body feel warm, cozy, and safe, such as warm milk, root vegetable soups, and hot cereals. Lightening qualities are catabolic. They reduce mass, reduce the tissues, eliminate excess water and mucus, and put a spring in your step. Lightening foods feel refreshing, enlivening, and energizing. Examples of lightening foods are steamed vegetables with lemon, bitter greens, clear soups, fresh melon, and ginger tea.

THE TEN BUILDERS AND THEIR OPPOSITES

NOTE: In translating the Sanskrit to English, sometimes it takes more than one English word to describe the felt quality. This is why some of the qualities enlist more than one word in the table that follows. You will also notice that some of the qualities result as much from *activities* (in italics in the table) as they do from substances ingested.

HEAVY: Heavy foods can feel like a brick or like a tonic in the body, depending on the way the food was prepared and the condition the digestive system is in when the substances come down the tube. Heavy foods digest best when they are taken warm and with a bit of spicing (imagine the opposite, the effect of a cold fondue). Examples: cow's cheese, fatty meats, saturated fats, *sedentary activities*.

LIGHT: A light quality makes you feel clearheaded and energetic.
Examples: foods that are easy to digest, like broth, raw vegetables, and fruits. Light quality is encouraged by *vigorous exercise* and *meditation*.

SLOW/DULL: Foods that digest slowly or make the body and mind dull carry this quality.
Examples: fried foods, beef, *overeating*, *oversleeping*.

SHARP/PENETRATING/QUICK: Think about foods that clear the sinus in a hurry, make your appetite sharp, or help you think straight.
Examples: wasabi, vinegar, pepper, ginger, alcohol, and sharp cheeses (including goat cheese).

COOL: A cool quality is introduced not only by foods that are cool when you eat them but also by foods that have a cooling effect. When you eat such foods, you are likely to feel cold or refreshed.
Examples: cilantro, cucumbers, limes, coconut.

HOT: Foods that are warm as well as foods with a heating effect introduce this quality into the body.
Examples: chilies, citrus, coffee, *smoking*, *practicing hot yoga*. Anything that has a propensity to cause acid indigestion will be heating.

OILY/UNCTUOUS: Humid weather can make you feel oily, as well as all oils and foods containing natural oils.
Examples: olive, coconut, sesame, and other oils; nuts, fish, seeds, olives.

DRY: A dry quality can appear in the mouth, skin, nose and throat, joints, or colon. Some foods absorb water from the body and contain little or no oil, giving them a drying effect. Some nondry substances may have been processed into a dry state; wheat, for instance, is not a dry grain, but refined and baked into crackers, it can be drying.
Examples: corn, large beans such as kidney and garbanzo, barley, rye, caffeine.

SMOOTH: A smooth quality feels soothing and mellow. Eating foods that feel smooth will smooth the skin as well as the intestines.
Examples: avocados, ripe mangoes, bananas, *swimming*.

ROUGH: Rough foods require lots of chewing.
Examples: corn chips, popcorn, coarse flours, celery sticks and other raw vegetables, *jogging in the cold*.

DENSE/SOLID: A dense quality may present as a heavy feeling in the head or entire body, lethargy, or sleepiness. Small volumes of dense foods will satisfy the appetite without creating imbalance. Too much at once, however, or dense foods taken at night can be difficult to digest.
Examples: cooked vegetables, cheeses, gluten, *sitting around*.

LIQUID: Density is diluted by a liquid quality. You can render a food less dense by watering it down, such as when you skim milk from cream. A food that has been liquefied—for instance, cooked into a soup—will have a less dense effect on the body.
Examples: broth, skim milk, lassi. *Sweating* will melt away dense quality.

SOFT: A soft quality makes the body and attitude gentle, supple, and moist. You can soften all foods by cooking and by adding liquid.
Examples: mashed potatoes, brie cheese, baked squash, fruit compote, *practicing gentle yoga*.

HARD: A hard quality makes the body stiff, dry, and aggressive. You can harden all foods by dehydrating and by consuming them in raw form.
Examples: corn, nuts, rye crackers, very crisp apples, grains and beans that aren't fully cooked, *competitive or aggressive forms of exercise*.

STABLE: A stable quality feels safe, comfortable, steady. Foods that increase a stable quality will be nourishing, low in sugar, and high in fat and protein. Salt increases a stable quality by helping the body to hold water.
Examples: meat, dairy products, miso, nuts, oils, *staying in one place*, *following a routine*.

MOBILE/UNSTABLE: A mobile quality can feel both inspiring and unsteady. It could show up as a healthy urge to travel or as hypermobile digestion (diarrhea). Foods that make the body clear, hot, and light increase a mobile quality; they are high in sugars that burn up quickly.
Examples: spicy dishes, raw foods, not enough food, juices, sugars, *travel*, or *relocating*.

CLOUDY/SLIMY: A cloudy quality in the body can feel like slow digestion or constipation, clogging of the pores, brain fog, or difficulty making decisions. A cloudy quality in foods manifests as opaque or translucent liquids, like creamy soups, fibrous fruits, and dark or yeasty beers. Ingestion of drugs, prescription or otherwise, and of alcohol increases a cloudy quality.

CLEAR: A clear quality can feel focused and light; it promotes complete bowel movements and clear skin. A clear quality is encouraged by foods that are clear, by *meditation* and *yoga*, and by *clean living*.
Examples: cucumbers and other watery vegetables, vegetable broth, herbal teas, plain water, *deep breathing*.

GROSS/BIG: *Gross* is a word used often in yoga. It means "of the physical body, the material world." The gross body includes all of our tissues, liquids, and wastes. Paying attention to the body without considering the soul or spirit will increase the gross quality and an individual's identification with the physical body only. Too much food, too much sleep, consumption of foods with too many building qualities will increase the gross quality.

SUBTLE/SMALL: A subtle quality refers to the energy vibration of the body, or *prana*. A subtle quality also suggests an awareness of the soul or spirit aspect of an individual. Eating freshly prepared, minimally processed, home-cooked foods, paying attention to the spiritual aspects of life, reading of spiritual or inspirational materials, and the *practice of yoga*, *healing arts*, and *meditation* will increase the subtle quality.

Certain qualities will be easy to notice, while others may seem elusive. One's awareness gets deeper with time, so just start by paying attention to the obvious and you will gradually get the hang of how your foods are affecting you.

Nature's Tool Kit: Using the Qualities in Your Cooking

Cold is one of the qualities, or properties, Ayurveda has designated to be used as a tool for encouraging balance. Its opposite is hot. The good news is there are only ten qualities and their ten opposites, a total of twenty tools you'll want to get to know. As you become sensitized to what these qualities feel like in your body and how they result from your food intake and activities, your intuitive choices for balance will begin to yield an autonomous sense of well-being. The twenty qualities will be referenced throughout the recipes to familiarize you with the foods that foster balance at different times of the year. Begin to think of these twenty attributes when you think about the Ayurvedic lifestyle. Take time as you eat your meals to notice how these qualities are present on your plate and in your body. Notice how you feel before and after exercise to see what qualities are manifesting: Clear or cloudy? Light or dense?

The shopping lists in the seasonal chapters will help you get organized to buy foods that balance the qualities of each season. This means the food you buy will have attributes opposite to those prevalent in the season.

BOTTOM LINE: Like increases like, so if you are feeling too hot, no matter the season, reduce foods with a heating effect and favor cooling foods from the summer chapter. If you often feel cold, introduce warming foods from the winter chapter and limit your intake of cold foods and drinks. Support your dietary choices by introducing activities that warm the body, like brisk walking. If you are accustomed to enjoying cold drinks, turn to the "Drinkables" sections in the fall and winter chapters to find some new recipe ideas (including warm smoothies—a delicious novelty).

THE SEASONS AND THEIR QUALITIES

Remember, the foods you will focus on in each season will have attributes opposite to those listed here, to foster balance.

SPRING: Heavy, oily/damp, slow, cloudy, stable	OPPOSITES: Light, dry, sharp, clear, mobile
SUMMER: Hot, sharp/bright, oily/humid	OPPOSITES: Cooling, slow/soft, dry
FALL: Cool, light, dry, rough, mobile/windy, clear	OPPOSITES: Warming, heavy, moist/oily, smooth, stable, cloudy/dense
WINTER: Cool, very dry, light, rough, hard, clear, mobile	OPPOSITES: Warming, moist/oily, heavy, smooth, soft, cloudy/dense, stable

The Six Tastes: Sensations of Our World

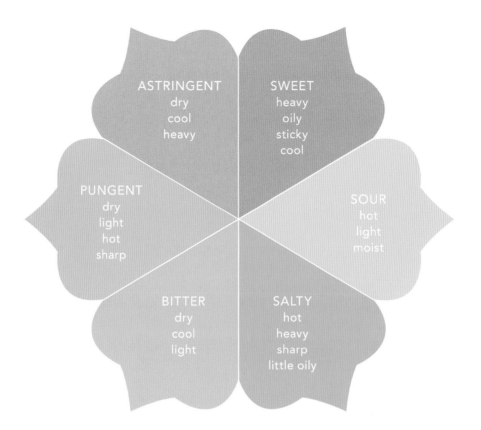

In the body, the twenty qualities naturally tend to gather in groups and get aggravated all together. Since sensing the qualities can be a rather subtle art, some people find the qualities are easier to recognize in a group. The groups are called "tastes," and the six tastes are another tool to help us integrate beneficial qualities through food choices. For example, foods that predominate in the heavy, oily, cool, and sticky qualities of water and earth elements will taste sweet, like dairy products. Foods that predominate in the dry, cool, light qualities of space and air will taste bitter, like kale.

Again, to get to know the tastes, rely on your body and your senses. The tongue will recognize a grouping of qualities as a certain taste, and a meal that contains all of the tastes is known to balance not only the palate but also the elements in the body. You might find you recognize taste more easily than individual qualities, especially at first, so learn about them here, and we will continue to grow familiar with the six tastes throughout the recipes.

Each taste results from the qualities of two elements combined.

MADHURA, SWEET TASTE, results from the qualities of earth and water (heavy, oily, sticky, cool). This taste creates a feeling of pleasure and comfort and signals food that builds strong bodily tissues (thanks to the structure of earth and the lubrication of water). By "sweet" I don't mean sugar here; think more of the natural sweetness inherent in grains (such as rice), in fruits, in root vegetables (potatoes, carrots, parsnips, beets), and in dairy products. Sugarcane and coconut sugar are also used in Ayurveda and in this book. White sugar is considered a poison to the body and thus something to be avoided.

Foods with sweet taste are especially good for the bones, skin, hair, and reproductive tissues, but in excess they can cause problems of fat tissue and diabetes.

AMLA, SOUR TASTE, results from the qualities of fire and earth (hot, light, moist). We can guess its effect will be heating, right? Sour taste makes the mouth water (water element), causes the teeth to tingle, and makes the eyes scrunch. You will recognize sour taste by the saliva coming into your mouth. Some sour foods are lemons, tart berries, most unripe fruits (including tomatoes), store-bought yogurt, pickles, tamarind, fermented foods, and vitamin C.

Sour taste stimulates the *agni*, digestive fire, which makes it a great taste in a condiment or appetizer. The light quality in sour taste cleanses and energizes the body's tissues and senses. In excess, the heat and wet of sour taste can cause irritation and swelling.

LAVANA, SALTY TASTE, results from the qualities of fire and water (hot, heavy, sharp, a little oily). Salt improves your power of taste by increasing saliva and makes everything taste better. Traditionally Ayurvedic cookery favors rock salt, but it has a strong sulphur flavor; in this book I use a lot of pink salt and sea salt. Salt taste is also present in seaweed (I use nori, dulse, and kombu in numerous recipes) and in some seafoods, especially oysters.

Foods with salty taste improve digestive activity as well as lubricate and clear obstructions of the digestive and other channels. In excess, salty taste can cause swelling, dry skin, and diminished strength.

TIKTA, BITTER TASTE, results from the qualities of ether and air (dry, cool, light). Bitter taste overrides the other tastes, might make you cringe, and is generally not a favorite, but in small amounts, you might crave it. Bitter taste is present in coffee, dark leafy greens like kale and collards, fenugreek seeds, and turmeric. But please don't take this as a green light for coffee! Leafy greens are a far less acidic way to get your bitter taste, without irritating the stomach and drying the intestines.

Bitter is the most lightening of the tastes. Foods with bitter taste reduce fat, manage blood sugar, clean the blood of toxins, improve digestion, and reduce moisture. However, in excess, bitter taste can dry you out, make you cold, and deplete the body.

KATU, PUNGENT (SPICY) TASTE, results from the qualities of fire and air (dry, light, hot, sharp). Pungent taste excites and makes the eyes, nose, and tongue water. Found mostly in spices, pungent taste appears in black and hot peppers, garlic, mustard, onion—a lot of the ingredients used to make food taste good. Foods with pungent taste help remove mucus and dry up fat; they also dilate the channels of the body and get things moving. In excess, the hot and sharp qualities of pungency can irritate the stomach, while the dry and light qualities can deplete the reproductive tissues.

KASHAYA, ASTRINGENT TASTE, results from the qualities of air and earth (dry, cool, and heavy). Astringent taste contracts the tissues. Think of things that make you pucker and suck the water out of your mouth, like cranberries, pomegranate seeds, tea, red wine, and honey. Think about skin care astringents such as witch hazel, which contracts the pores. Astringency makes it harder for your palate to taste because it contracts your taste buds.

Foods with astringent taste tone any areas that may be slack, watery, or fatty, and they clean the blood. In excess, astringency can make you stiff, constipated, and thirsty.

The name of the game is moderation, of course. This is why Ayurveda is well known for encouraging the balanced inclusion of all six tastes in the diet. Look to the seasonal chutneys and spice blends to round out your flavors and in so doing round out your qualities, too.

The Seasonal Affect: Your Annual Cycles

It's all about the weather. The external conditions you are exposed to greatly affect whether your body is warm, cool, oily, dry, and so on. So much so that simply eating a diet that helps to balance the effects of the weather can be all it takes to allow your body to do its thing—that is, to keep healthy.

Rtucharya means "seasonal regimen." Simply eating the recipes from the seasonal chapters will get you started on this aspect of the Ayurvedic lifestyle. Changing your foods with the weather keeps you well. You don't have to memorize the following information or intellectually understand the changes—you need to feel for them in your annual cycles. Ayurveda's description of the seasonal affects provides a language to describe seasonal changes and to guide us into feeling the qualities of the natural world that affect us. If it doesn't make sense today, it's OK! Keep noticing and feeling—that's the Ayurvedic lifestyle.

Traditionally, Ayurveda recognized six seasons, because the weather of the Indian subcontinent sees varying levels of heat, cold, and moisture, including monsoons. For our purposes in the West, we identify four seasons, this way:

SPRING: Cool and damp

SUMMER: Hot and humid

FALL: Cooling and increasingly dry

WINTER: Cold and dry

If your seasons don't follow the same pattern described here—a wet and cool spring, then a hot and humid summer, followed by a dry fall, leading into a cold and dry winter—please see "Adapting for Different Climates" (page 67).

Here's how an annual cycle changes . . .

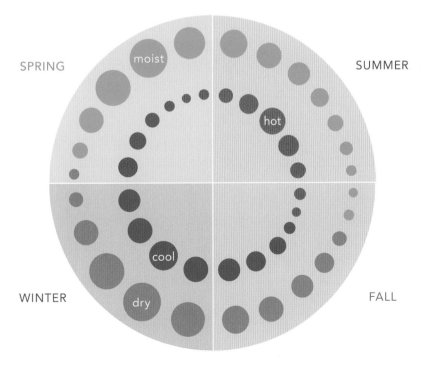

In spring, the environment is cool as it emerges from winter, but now winter's dryness gives way to damp. As the thaw begins and rains come, the body no longer needs thick mucus to protect it, and the mucus begins to melt. Just as the sap runs in maple trees, the body produces an unctuous, slow, cloudy liquid in need of reduction. Reactions to this cool, damp time of year may look like sinus and chest congestion, loss of appetite, sluggish digestion, lethargy, and/or sadness.

The tastes that balance spring are pungent, bitter, and astringent. Pungency warms, melts, and mobilizes; bitter and astringent tastes lighten and reduce excess moisture. Reduce building foods, be sure to exercise, and eat only when hungry.

In summer, the weather increasingly warms and may be wet. Keeping the body cool becomes important as the summer gets on. Reactions to hot and humid qualities (oily, penetrating, mobile) may look like acne, inflammatory conditions, swelling, acid stomach, and/or irritability.

The tastes that balance summer are bitter, sweet, and astringent. Sweet and bitter tastes have a cooling effect, and bitterness and astringency help reduce water in the body.

In the early fall, the body contains accumulated heat from the summer and is experiencing increasing dryness with the coming winds, which aggravates the internal heat. Reactions to the combination of heat and dryness may present as itchy or burning rashes, loose stools, dandruff, acid stomach, dry eye, and/or unstable emotions.

As late fall comes on, the heat subsides, and the body feels cold and dry. The late fall is really the beginning of winter, a time to transition. The appetite gets stronger, and it is the period to begin building.

The tastes that balance early fall are bitter, astringent, and sweet. Bitter and sweet tastes reduce heat, while astringency sucks excess water from the summer out of the body and pulls it down and out. The tastes that balance late fall are salty, sweet, and sour—same as for winter. All of these tastes warm and moisturize the body, because of their composition of fire, earth, and water elements.

In the winter, dry and cold qualities accumulate. The increase of building qualities (dense, oily, warm, smooth, and so forth) protects the body from the cold, and you will experience an increase and thickening of the mucous membranes (in the sinuses, lungs, and intestines) to protect your system from the dry quality, which will only increase until the thaw in spring. A reaction to the combination of cold and dry could look like constipation, brittle or stiff feelings in the joints or bones, anxiety, and/or weight gain.

As the late winter comes on, the body maxes out on building and mucus-producing qualities, the appetite decreases, the digestion slows down, and it is time to begin introducing a bit of lighter foods–but serve them warm.

The tastes to balance winter are sweet, sour, and salty, for their building and moisturizing qualities. The addition of more pungent taste in the late winter will begin to lighten the body and sharpen the digestive fire.

In Ayurveda the effect the seasonal variations have on the body is important enough to be named as one of the three main causes of imbalance.

SEASONAL CLEANSING

Ayurveda recommends a light diet at the change of seasons, most important, spring and fall, and a healthy, balancing cleanse routine. In the spring, the body needs to expel excess mucus accumulated during winter, while in the fall, the body needs to expel heat accumulated during the summer. Getting rid of stuff is something the body is good at, provided you keep an eye on what's going in. Practices like eating simply, reducing foods that feed the accumulation of the past season, and having a bit of rest gently ensure that the body has an opportunity to recalibrate and head into the next half of the year in top form. See Seasonal Cleansing (Seasonal Self-Care) for easy-to-follow guidelines.

How Do We Get Out of Whack?

THE THREE CAUSES OF IMBALANCE

Ayurveda recognizes three main causes of disease and imbalance, called *trividha karana*. If the human being manages these three areas well, the body should remain in a state of relative balance, and the progression from imbalance to disease will not occur.

The three factors are:

- *KALA:* Time of day and time of year (seasonal affect)
- *ARTHA:* Too much or too little use of the sense organs
- *KARMA:* Actions and activities pertaining to body, speech, and mind,[2] which includes *prajnaparadha*, crimes against wisdom

KALA: THE SEASONAL AFFECT

The organization of recipes and seasonal discernment in this book is intended to balance the seasonal affect. If you are new to Ayurveda, all you need to know is that if you follow the big lunch/small supper principle, make seasonal food choices, and observe a bit of lifestyle routine, you will lower your risk of getting sick at the change of seasons. Think about it: spring and fall, the major junctures in weather changes, are the times when many people become ill with colds, flus, and allergies. This book will get you cooking with a sense of what the seasonal diet is all about and get you tasting your way through the annual cycle. I'll bet you feel better, sharing in nature's routine.

The effects of seasonal variation can cause the body to go out of balance. The need to keep warm in fall after trying to keep cool all summer, for example, can knock the body for a loop. If one is paying attention and responding to the changing qualities of the season—for instance, by shifting to warm, oily foods as the weather gets cool and dry in the fall—one can avoid problems caused by excessive cool and dry qualities coming suddenly into the body, such as dry skin, constipation, or cold hands and feet. A traditionally practiced monodiet at the change of seasons, as described in the spring and fall cleanse sections (see pages 298–99), also assists the body in adjusting.

ARTHA: MISUSE OF THE SENSE ORGANS

The sense organs are the body parts responsible for the five senses: ears (hearing), eyes (sight), tongue (taste), skin (touch), and nose (smell). Misuse can mean too much stimulation of the senses as well as too little. The nervous system is taxed by digesting too much information from the sense organs. The sense organ itself may begin to suffer, such as when you have red, dry, itchy eyes after too much screen time or when your tongue builds up a tolerance to salty restaurant food and you feel the need to increase your use of salt. Bringing the senses back into balance settles the nervous system, thereby reducing stress, which is often the cause of imbalance in the first place. For example, if people who have trouble sleeping limit their TV, smartphone, or computer time at night, they are more likely to enjoy a good night's rest.

Usually the problem lies in exposing the senses to too much stimulation. Here are a few general suggestions to reduce strain on the sense organs.

Ears. Go easy on the iPod and take a break sometimes. Silence works wonders. Notice the qualities of the music you do choose to listen to and check in with yourself: is it appropriate for the time of day and your mental state? Music that is too upbeat may give you difficulty sleeping, while music containing angry lyrics might exacerbate your irritation.

Eyes. As mentioned, limit computer, smartphone, and TV time as much as possible. Track your screen activity and notice how much time per day feels appropriate for you and at what point your eyes need a break. Rest the eyes by closing them and taking a few deep breaths from time to time. If this proves difficult, try using an eye pillow, lying down with it set gently over your eyes to block out the light for a few minutes.

Tongue: Stick to natural, unrefined foods without added flavors, white sugars, or too much salt. Acclimate your taste buds to the lighter sensations of foods in their natural form. Practice right speech; notice how much you talk from day to day and whether you tend to criticize. With a little practice, quietude becomes calming.

Skin: Oil the skin daily to quiet the nerve endings. Favor natural oils, such as sesame, coconut, and almond, over conventional moisturizers. Dress warmly when needed.

Nose: Reduce your use of products containing "fragrance." Note that cutting down on onion and garlic in your diet will lessen your need for deodorant.

MODERATING MEDIA AND CONNECTIVITY

It is not necessary to be available to everybody all the time. Productivity is not the only aim of this life. Turn off the phone and e-mail sometimes and enjoy the quiet pleasures of the senses as you bring your awareness to the slant of light in the room, the colors of the world around you, the warmth and flavor of a sip of herbal tea. Get outside, shift your attention away from the internal chatter of the mind, and observe the larger world.

You may have heard a lot of this before and dismissed it in the movements of daily life. It's easy to scoff at suggestions regarding slants of light and herbal tea. However, a sense of balance will be elusive until we learn to shift our attention from our to-do list or the broken-record sounds of stress to the sweetness of engaging the senses with our world. Changing old patterns takes practice, and the first step on the path is the desire to change.

Karma and Prajnaparadha: Crimes against Wisdom

Karma means "action." Not necessarily good or bad, just action. Every action produces a reaction. Choosing a certain meal to eat, for example, is an action. How that meal affects your body is the reaction. According to classical Ayurveda texts, acting to suppress natural urges, such as going to the bathroom or having a good cry, can cause imbalance. The action of suppression causes a reaction over time, resulting in imbalance. Our own actions—or inactions—can get us in a pickle!

Prajnaparadha means "crimes against wisdom"—in other words, knowing what the right thing to do is but doing the opposite anyway. Why do we choose ice cream over herbal tea? Making the choice that harms instead of helps appears to be a tendency of human nature; indeed, we seem to have been doing it for at least a few millennia, according to the Ayurveda texts. Actions such as going back for seconds on dessert when you are full or staying up late when you are tired are two of those things we do knowing full well it's not a good idea. In the beginning, turning a more aware eye to your choices, you're likely to watch yourself commit a few crimes. It happens! Take heart, and remember that with practice you will see that making a healthy choice actually creates a positive reaction. After experiencing a few positive reactions, the healthy choice becomes more appealing.

Note that when the body is in a state of imbalance, cravings are likely to reflect that imbalance. For instance, someone with too much heat in the body might crave foods that increase heat. The imbalance itself begins to do the talking. When the body comes back toward its state of balance, the cravings will subside. For now, simply follow the general seasonal guidelines in this book to encourage states of balance. From there, you might notice certain cravings diminish without your having to think too hard about it.

What Do Balance and Imbalance Look Like?

Luckily, Ayurveda has described early signs of imbalance to help us know when we are getting off-kilter. But keep in mind, we are not all on the same axis to begin with, and some of the points listed here may never be in balance for you all the time. Imbalance is nothing to beat yourself up about. You can think of these signs as a heads-up, to help you recognize early symptoms of imbalance that can be sorted out with diet and lifestyle awareness.

Watch out for:
- Constipation (not having a bowel movement every day)
- Gas and bloating after meals
- Excessively dry skin, burning or itching sensations
- Cold hands and feet
- Frequent burping, acid indigestion
- Hot flashes or profuse sweating
- Swelling

- Loss of appetite
- Congestion
- Insomnia

In a state of relative balance, you can expect to enjoy:
- A daily bowel movement first thing in the morning, one that is well formed, floating, and about the size, shape, and texture of a ripe banana
- No bloating after meals
- Consistent, hearty appetite
- Sound sleep, so you wake feeling refreshed
- Clear complexion
- Comfortable body temperature
- Easy breathing

To further help you prevent imbalance, Ayurveda tells us that disease can arise from habitually suppressing or forcing the following natural urges:

- Eliminating feces
- Urinating
- Releasing gas
- Sneezing
- Vomiting
- Thirst
- Hunger
- Sleep
- Coughing
- Breathing
- Yawning

Agni, Prana, and *Ojas*: Fostering Digestion, Energy, and Immunity

These three concepts are the keys to vibrant health. Supporting the digestive fire, keeping the energy circulating smoothly, and protecting our vital essence comprise the foundational trinity of Ayurvedic practice.

AGNI (UG-NEE)

Agni is a word you might recognize. It means "fire," one of the five elements. When it comes to digestion, *agni* refers to *jathara agni*, the fire of the stomach. The classic texts of Ayurveda open with information on agni. Keeping the digestive fire strong is the number-one priority. If one has the correct amounts of water, fire, space, and food in the stomach, one should digest food well, meaning the stomach makes a nice ahara rasa, juice of the food. As mentioned earlier, the juice of the food is the building block of healthy tissues.

When agni is burning strongly, toxicity is not allowed to lodge in the tissues; rather, it breaks down and is eliminated. In this way, good digestive fire keeps the body free of *ama*, undigested matter, which gunks up the works, weakens the system, and promotes imbalance. The health, stamina, and luster of your body begin right in your stomach.

The jathara agni in the stomach builds like a little campfire. You must have kindling to get it started. If you put too much wood on it, the fire is smothered. If you don't give it enough wood, the fire can't burn strongly enough to create light and warmth.

Smothering the fire by overeating is a common cause of low agni and is easily remedied by skipping a meal to allow the fire to build up again (except in the case of eating disorders or unsteady blood-sugar levels). Any time you feel a loss of appetite, this indicates that you have a low digestive fire, and it's a good time to skip a meal.

Ayurvedic cookery uses spices as kindling to build agni. For example, eating a small amount of fresh ginger before a meal will make you feel hungry, because adding kindling increases your fire.

GETTING TO KNOW YOUR DIGESTIVE FIRE

Start by feeling for your agni. Get familiar with the fire in the stomach by noticing when you are hungry and what your hunger feels like. And learn to differentiate between the hunger of the stomach and the hunger of the tongue. The tongue wants stuff that tastes good, while the stomach wants stuff that will steadily make building blocks for health and vitality. To tell the difference, ask yourself: Is it only oatmeal chocolate chip cookies that sound good right now, or would I get excited to eat a big plate of steamed vegetables? I think you see where I am going with this . . .

Getting to know your digestive fire is really that simple!

The amount of water to take at a meal is specified as about one-third of the size of the stomach (think about four to six ounces). This leaves a third of your stomach for food and a third for space and air to move it around. Some of the water might be included in your food, such as a soupy stew or a watery vegetable like a cucumber. The correct amount of water ensures your digestive system makes a nice juice of the food. Quality oil, especially ghee, is considered the best lighter fluid and helps the fire reduce the food into juice. Ayurveda recommends about one teaspoon per meal.

Throughout the digestive process, the jathara agni is followed by little fires, breaking down fats and proteins, metabolizing, absorbing, and making body tissues like fats and muscles. This metabolizing process is governed by *tejas*, the bright, energetic essence of fire and metabolic activity.

Fired up to boost your agni? Delve into chapter 2 to get to work.

Remember this: eating when you are truly hungry and eating slowly enough to sense when you begin to feel full are all you really need to do to care for your digestive fire. These simple practices can ensure the health, luster, and stamina you are looking for.

PRANA (PRAAH-NAH)

Prana, meaning something like "vital energy" or "life energy," has become a bit of a buzzword. Those meanings are correct—but it also means so much more. Prana is the energy of life. An organism without prana is dead. Your body without prana is only a mash-up of the five elements—there's nothing moving.

But here's a key fact, and what fascinates me about how the ancient science of Ayurveda is reeducating us: where the attention goes, the prana follows. The life energy is a servant of the mind. This means it is ever so important to focus on the food we are eating.

Preparing our own food, taking care with how we buy it, eating it with our full attention—all the way from the shopping to the cooking to the eating, we have opportunities to increase the life energy of our foods and thus the energy we receive by eating them. If you want to feel good, pay attention!

Culturally, mealtimes tend to have a lot of focal points other than the food. Here are a few tips to build the prana potential of your meals.

Reduce mixing *eating* with *meeting*. That's actually a slogan of mine. When I have a request for a working lunch, I suggest a teatime instead. Or else I have a quiet, square meal earlier or later that day, which frees me up to eat more lightly and depend less on that working meal for nourishment, since the attention is meant to go to the business at hand, not to the acts of eating and digesting.

Talk about the food. If you are enjoying a social or family meal, you might find the food is being served and no one even notices. Try remarking on the glorious colors, aromas, and tastes of the dishes being shared. Your enthusiasm might encourage your companions to join you in a moment of reflection. Even if the attention moves away later, try to begin the digestive process with appreciation and attention for the food.

Take three deep breaths before eating. Filling the abdominal region with breath brings prana to that area. This will help prepare the body to receive the food.

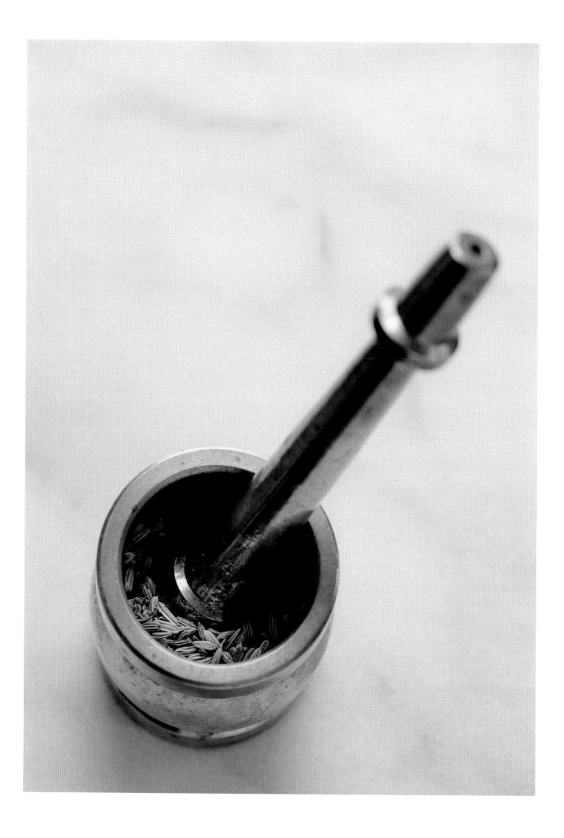

OJAS (OH-JOS)

Ojas is the subtle essence of our life energy. Unlike prana, which is a movement or vibration of energy, ojas is a substance. You might think of it as the cream of the body, the richest and most nourishing stuff.

The Charaka Samhita[3] describes ojas as that "which keeps all the living beings refreshed."[4] Ayurveda suggests human beings have a limited, predetermined amount of ojas. Living too large burns ojas. You arrive on earth with a full tank. If you put the pedal to the metal, you will burn the fuel up faster. *Poof* goes your longevity—and, along the way, your immunity.

In my home city of Boston, I see a lot of people who get out of bed, leave the house immediately, work all day without a lunch break, eat a big dinner, then go to bed. A lifestyle that consistently doesn't leave time for the body to be nourished at midday is one way to force the body to burn its reserves. Living in fear or stress is another. Slowing the pace a bit, respecting the limitations of the body, and in general *doing less* will preserve ojas.

Did she say "doing less"? It's not the global lifestyle norm these days. Even so, this is one of the main messages of Ayurveda. Humans have come to expect to operate at a ceaseless pace of forward, march! Consider that this may not be a sustainable practice.

One can build ojas and along with it the body's immunity. This book contains a few ojas-building recipes (see sidebar above). Ojas builders are rich foods, with warming spices to help the body digest them, and should be taken with full attention in limited quantities at the appropriate time. In fact, certain ojas-building foods are revered for their connection to our vital essence, such as dates, almonds, milk, and ghee. These foods are always offered at ceremonies in Hindu temples.

Now that you have some background on Ayurveda, let's get down to the real nitty-gritty: the Ayurvedic eating concept.

OJAS-BUILDING RECIPES

Everyday Ghee (page 120)
Hemp Protein Squares (page 174)
Saffron Lassi (page 282)
Spiced Nut Milk Smoothie (page 235)
Stuffed Dates (page 277)
Winter Rejuvenating Tonic (page 279)

CHAPTER 2

The Principles of Ayurvedic Eating

Ayurvedic cookery is more than just what you whip up in the kitchen—it's a whole way of life. The recipe section of this book will guide you into an Ayurvedic diet and lifestyle. The recipes themselves are suggestions to get you started, but what this book really aims to do is to teach you how to integrate Ayurvedic principles into both your cooking and your daily life. The concept includes preparing fresh food for yourself, eating in a seasonal rhythm, and enjoying consistent mealtimes. What follows are pointers to help you attend to aspects of your diet that aren't as much about the foods themselves as they are about the overall role food is playing in your life.

Ayurvedic eating takes into account intention and attitude, time of day, whether something is a meal versus a snack, portion size, the season, and the dining space. In this chapter you will find a practice tip for each of these aspects so that you can start experimenting with new ideas about food. To ensure success, begin with the one or two that speak to you, rather than trying to engage all the tips at once. Easing into change keeps the body/mind stable, while trying to accomplish too much too fast can result in a burnout.

If Habit Is Driving, Stop the Car

The work of forging new habits takes discipline in the beginning, but once in motion, it gets easier, and eventually the new practices become second nature. In fact, the hardest part might be recognizing your old patterns and changing how you do things. Imagine that you are driving in the mud over the same route again and again, so the tire tracks begin to get deep and it becomes difficult to get out. The first steps to creating fresh tracks are to stop the car, back it up, and start again in a new direction. In the moment a craving or habit pattern comes up, pause, take a breath, and ask yourself what action will help you feel better in the long run. With a little awareness, you will become awake enough to stop the car before you go down the same old path. Now on the fresh track, the driving gets easier, and you are more likely to arrive where you intend to go.

The practice tips below offer actions for change, because old habits need new ones to take their place. Again, you don't have to act on them all; just start by paying attention to the following aspects of your food world.

Booby Trap Alert! When you're forging new habits, you might experience a lag time between noticing the old, nonbeneficial habit and changing the accustomed action to one that's better for you. This can be tough on your heart. Take a breath and be kind to yourself. Remember, humans have been working on living well for thousands of years. Giving yourself a hard time can set you up to feel unsatisfied, incompetent, and then defeated. Celebrate your growing awareness with the affirmation that you are in a process. Know that simply noticing the old patterns is the first step toward change—and it can be the hardest step. Before making your move, give yourself a preemptive pat on the back.

The Why, How, How Much, When, and Where of Eating

WHY AND HOW WE EAT

In Ayurveda, *why* we eat is the most important factor in our relationship to food, as it determines how the food will be received by the body. When you begin to use food as medicine, hold the intention for the food to be nourishing, energizing, enjoyable, and easy on your body. Keep in mind, there is room for both enjoyment and nourishment. Ayurveda references the hunger of the tongue as well as the hunger of the stomach. Pleasing the palate is an important aspect of Ayurvedic cookery, one that is accomplished through the use of digestive spices and the inclusion of the six tastes (see page 18).

Eating foods that one dislikes is not considered beneficial. So, although the focus is on nourishment first, remember that the foods you eat should also be pleasing to you.

How we eat is certainly more important than what we eat. For instance, you could have a carefully chosen, lovingly prepared meal in front of you, but if you eat it while worrying that it will cause you to gain weight, the worry can create nervous indigestion or cause your body to reject the food.

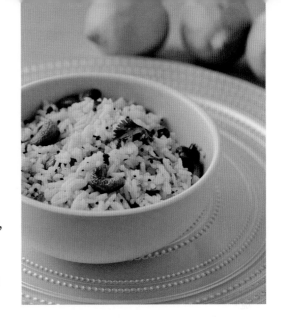

The key to eating with the right mind-set is to approach your meals with gratitude. Just as you would take care to listen to a friend in need, take care to notice your foods. As soon as your body smells food, it begins to prepare the appropriate enzymes for the fare it recognizes. Before you've even taken a bite into your mouth, the process of digestion has begun! Engage the senses by looking closely, smelling, and feeling the qualities of the food on your plate. What colors, scents, and textures do you observe?

PRACTICE TIP: Make a practice of taking a few moments to sit with the food before you eat it—just a few breaths to take it all in with your senses and to prepare for eating.

HOW MUCH?

Imagine that your stomach is divided into four parts. The ancient texts of Ayurveda suggest that "two parts of the stomach should be filled with solid foods, one part by liquids, and the remaining one part should be kept vacant for accommodating air."[1] The amount of solid food you can hold in your cupped hands is a good measure to go by.

Drinking liquid is an important part of each meal. The ideal drink would be warm water, plain or with fresh-squeezed lemon, or a digestive tea, which you will find recipes for in the seasonal sections of this book. A small cup of six ounces or so will suffice. Drinking a lot of water less than thirty minutes before a meal or within two hours afterward will dilute the digestive juices. The right amount of liquid will make a nice ahara rasa, juice of the food.

WHEN WE EAT

Eating at the proper time of day determines whether the food will be well digested or not. Believe it or not, a burger at noon is preferable to a salad at midnight. In Ayurveda what we are working toward is to eat food at mealtimes and nothing in between. The general recommendation is three meals a day, but for some people, two meals a day may be enough; others may need four. This will depend on your amount of physical activity, your particular metabolism, and, of course, the season—in the winter, for example, you are likely to be hungrier than in the summer and eat more to keep your body warm.

Remember that the digestive fire is like a campfire. If you wait too long to add wood to it, the fire will die out. If you continuously add wood to it, you will smother the flames, and you will need to stop adding and wait until it grows again before putting more wood on. Most of us are in the habit of eating too often. The fire never gets to come to full strength because it always has something new to digest. The practice of not eating between meals allows the fire to grow.

Once you feel comfortable with your breakfast and lunch routine, you can start observing how much food you need to eat at lunchtime to keep you from getting too hungry or spacey before dinner. At the very least, you will begin noticing if you have a tendency to skimp at lunchtime and end up eating a few other things (like sweets and coffee) through the afternoon. A full lunch will keep you satisfied and out of trouble.

It took me about six months to feel comfortable eating only at mealtimes. One day I was so hungry after breakfast and the next I was stuffed! I hadn't been in the habit of eating meals—I was a grazer, and it all felt new to me. After a year, I felt like eating only at mealtimes and I experienced fewer symptoms of poor digestion by allowing each meal to completely digest. Even so, some days I say forget it, and I have a snack! I take pleasure in indulging in a break from the routine from time to time.

NOTE: The metabolism needs time to get used to a shift in eating patterns. Take care not to be too rigid about it and give yourself plenty of time to transition to eating square meals at routine times of day. If you make it happen even half of the time, you are doing your digestion a favor.

TRUE HUNGER

Hungry? Are you sure about that? Get in the habit of noticing before you eat something: How strong is the hunger? Know that about two hours after a meal (maybe more if it's a big one), the stomach opens the trapdoor and the food moves down from the stomach into the small intestine. The stomach has suddenly gone from full to empty, and you'll feel a sensation of emptiness there—but if you ate just two hours ago, it's unlikely you're experiencing true hunger. Wait. In a half hour or less, you won't feel hungry anymore, and your body will begin to harness the energy from the food you are still digesting. True hunger gets stronger if you wait an hour, and you get to the next meal with a healthy fire. Watch for this hunger pattern about two hours after a meal, and you will begin to recognize it for what it is.

Remember, if you feel hungry for a cookie, but switching to thoughts of vegetable soup doesn't really get your fires going, it is your tongue that is hungry and not your stomach. Allow yourself to get truly hungry, and you will crave more beneficial foods.

Suggested Daily Rhythm

The heat of the digestive fire mirrors the heat of the sun as it warms up and cools down over the course of the day. The following meal schedules optimize digestion, supported by this natural flow.

Breakfast. Before noon, the fire has not yet reached its peak. Try a light breakfast to ease you into the day, though if you are awake early or exercise before breakfast, you may find the morning meal needs to be more substantial. Eat enough to get you through to lunch.

Big Lunch. As the sun reaches its peak after noon, lunch is the ideal time to eat the largest amount of food and/or the most complex foods, such as fats and proteins. It is also the time for eating one of those treats someone brought into the office today, rather than snacking on it between meals.

Supper. The word *supper* is similar to the word *supplement.* This light evening meal is meant to supplement your food intake if you didn't get enough food earlier in the day. If you are in the habit, as many are, of having a family or social meal at night, do yourself a favor by being sure to eat a good lunch. You will be less tempted to overeat in the evening, the time when the digestive system is winding down for the day. Remember that family and social meals can be more about the precious time you spend with your loved ones than about the food. Shift your focus to being nourished by the company you are with, and you will feel satisfied by a lighter meal.

Eating dinner two to three hours before bedtime ensures that you fall asleep without food still in your stomach. This will allow your organs to perform some cleanup while you rest, rather than having to work through that late dinner you ate. As in all things Ayurveda, it's what you do habitually that counts. It's fine to have late meals sometimes, but as a general habit, eat lightly and early.

Another daily rhythm, one that works well in hot weather, is to take two meals a day: a bigger meal in the late morning, before the temperature gets too warm, and a more modest one as the day cools down, before the sun sets. In hot countries, people characteristically take a siesta in the afternoon and eat a late supper, after dark, when it is cool. In the American

YOU DESERVE A LUNCH BREAK

I run into this conflict all the time: a nine-to-fiver in the city looks at me like I'm nuts when I suggest she leave her desk for thirty minutes to take lunch or even turn around so her chair faces a window or go outside to sit on a bench. Who decided you don't get a lunch break? *You.* Although in your workplace you may feel pressure to shove food in your mouth while working, this doesn't mean you aren't entitled, by law, to a break. Peer pressure is no reason to compromise your health. Eating while working *does* compromise your health. I draw a hard line here because I have seen a number of people find success and balance their health through a slow and steady commitment to taking lunch breaks. These are people who were resistant to the idea in the beginning, but upon experiencing the important benefits of the midday meal, they have successfully created a new habit!

latitudes, summer sunset may be as late as 9 P.M., so take the second meal around 5:00 or 6:00 if you plan to get to bed early.

WHAT WE EAT

What we eat is the aspect of diet everyone talks about, yet it is only a part of the whole picture in Ayurveda. The foods to eat are ones that balance the qualities of the season or the qualities you are experiencing at the time. The seasonal diet in this book ensures that you will get to enjoy all the tastes but at the appropriate times of year. The beauty of nature is that it provides us with foods that are beneficial for the season, like yams with their building qualities in winter and cilantro with its cooling qualities in summer.

> **PRACTICE TIP:** During each season, focus on the qualities presented in the beginning of that section in the book. Over the course of the year, you will have plenty of time to experience all twenty qualities as they emerge.

WHERE WE EAT

The place where one takes meals is most beneficial if it is quiet and peaceful, without too much sensory stimulation, such as loud music, talking, TV, computers, or strong artificial fragrances such as air freshener or perfume.

Sit down when you eat. Eating at your desk or on the run means you are eating while focusing on other activities. This habit will steal the energy from your digestive organs, leaving meals not fully digested or nutrients not fully absorbed, and it's unacceptable. Consider drawing a hard line with your schedule: set aside twenty to thirty minutes solely for eating your meal, and do not habitually use the mealtime to accomplish other tasks.

TAKING IT TO WORK

At work, the key to successful balanced eating is to be prepared. Purchase a lunch bag and a few sizes of glass Tupperware dishes that will hold enough food for your midday meals—not too much—and fit together in the bag. You might also want a small container for soaked almonds, toasted seeds, or other mix-ins. Cold food is harder to digest, so don't keep the bag in the fridge at work. Some dishes you may want to warm up by stirring in a bit of hot water. Microwaving destroys the pranic value of your foods, so when you can, bring your hot food to work in a thermos. Get in the habit of rinsing your lunch containers right after you eat or soon after you get home to avoid piling up dishes.

Traditional Tips for Improving Digestion

Following a few rules of thumb can make a huge difference in helping you maintain a healthy digestive fire, strong metabolism, and regular elimination. Some of these recommendations may seem simple, but the effects can be profound. Pay attention as you read the list below and see if one or two items jump out at you. Start by working on just those habits.

- Do not take iced drinks, especially with meals. Ask for hot or room-temperature tap or still bottled water at restaurants.
- Drink warm water throughout the day, and in cool weather carry a thermos instead of a water bottle.
- Favor warm, cooked foods over raw.
- Reduce the amount of leftovers you eat and get into the habit of cooking fresh meals more often.
- Wait two hours after meals before drinking.
- Space out your meals by at least three to four hours to allow for complete digestion before eating again. You may have to make this change gradually to allow your blood sugar to adjust. Avoid grazing–your digestive fire can never build up with constant input.
- Do not eat when you aren't hungry. It is OK to skip a meal if you're not hungry, and in fact it can be harmful to habitually eat when not hungry, even if the mind tells you it's time. Remember that sometimes you have to slow down to notice if you are truly in need of food.
- Take your time to eat and rest a little for ten minutes afterward, but do not sleep directly after eating.
- Take a light walk after you eat.
- If you are going to have a treat, enjoy it with lunch, when the digestion is strongest, and do not eat again until dinner.

Kindling Digestive Fire and Improving Assimilation: *Deepana* and *Pachana*

Special culinary spices are prized for their power to kick-start the appetite (*deepana*) and to improve the digestion of food and breakdown of *ama* (*pachana*). While the best way to reduce ama is to follow the aforementioned guidelines, any Ayurvedic diet will also make moderate use of digestive spices to support a clean burning system. The great news is these are all things you are likely to have in your kitchen already, like ginger, lemon, and black pepper.

You will find deepana and pachana substances most helpful when you are experiencing:

- a weak appetite
- a heavy feeling in the stomach
- a heavy feeling upon waking up
- a sleepy feeling after eating
- taking more than two hours to digest a meal
- trouble digesting a full meal

DEEPANA: Before a meal, try one of these two options to stimulate a sluggish appetite.

SPICY BEVERAGE

Into a full cup of warm water, add the fresh-squeezed juice of ¼–½ lemon and a hearty dash of black pepper. Drink this 20–30 minutes before a meal. You will get hungry!

GINGER BLASTER

Cut and peel a slice of gingerroot about ¼ inch thick and squeeze 1 tsp or so of lemon juice on it. Add a dash of salt. Chew 20–30 minutes before a meal.

PACHANA: After a meal, to alleviate bloating, gas, heavy stomach, and lethargy, try one of the following:

Make a strong cup of ginger tea, relax, and sip slowly.

Enjoy a digestive tea (see seasonal chapters for recommended recipes).

Get specific for your ailment: make one of the following teas by boiling 1 tsp of the spice or herb, whole or freshly ground, in 1 cup of water for 10–15 minutes.

- For acid stomach, fennel or mint tea.
- For bloating, ginger and turmeric tea.
- For a congested feeling, ginger and cumin tea.
- For sugar cravings, cinnamon tea.

NOTE: Do not use concentrated lemon juice; it does not have the same digestive qualities as fresh lemon.

The Flow of Food: Establishing a Rhythm

All the processes in your body that move do so in rhythm. The beat of your heart, the daily sleep cycle, the monthly hormonal cycles are all following a pattern. These rhythms are inherent. However, sometimes your external life becomes arrhythmic, meaning there is no pattern to your days. You might often go to sleep at 3 A.M. and at 9 P.M. a lot of the time, too, and sleep in until all different hours. You may not be able to say when you eat lunch most days; maybe you don't even get around to it sometimes and you don't notice.

The digestive system is like a pet dog. The dog gets in the habit of you coming in the door at 6 P.M. and feeding him. If you come home late or forget to feed him, he is going to get confused, hungry, and scared. The same thing happens when humans override the natural appetite and fail to eat meals on time. Inconsistencies in the timing of meals will create inconsistency of digestion and elimination, production of blood sugar, and mood swings.

Unlike the pet dog, in humans the mix-up happens gradually and is easy to ignore. But, like the dog, the digestion can be trained. If you make a point to be rhythmic about when you eat your meals, your bodily processes will run smoothly. The appetite and the acids and enzymes in the gut will get in the habit of building at the appropriate times of day, resulting in increased assimilation and absorption of nutrition. You will get more out of your food, need to eat less, and crave fewer nonbeneficial foods. You will feel better because rhythm is something the nerves can count on, and consistent mealtimes really help lower stress levels and diminish mood swings.

You just learned the suggested daily rhythm for meals, based on the rhythms nature dictates. This is an ideal to aim for, but not everyone is in a position to follow the ideal flow. Here are some more options to help you establish a healthy groove.

GIMME A BREAK

Remember, the rhythm points act as touchstones throughout the day. If you can make the suggested daily rhythm happen more often than not—say, four or five days a week—you can be proud of a job well done. Relaxing around your routines from time to time and indulging in free-form fun keeps you spontaneous and resilient—everybody needs a break from the routine. The best time to eat is when you are feeling good, not anxious or angry.

The Rhythm Project

The word *project* implies that finding a rhythm in your meal schedule is going to take some work. On Day 1, the change can be daunting. I have broken down the process into the following steps, based on what has worked for me and for my clients. Commit to the project for a few weeks, long enough to notice an improvement in how you feel. Feeling good will inspire you to keep going. As always, take it one step at a time, because Ayurveda teaches that small changes are lasting ones.

Start by carving out one consistent pattern in your eating schedule by finding a window for your morning meal, midday meal, or evening meal. (If you can, make it midday.) Practice eating a meal during that window most days for a week or two.

The next goal is to make this meal be one you prepare. This requires that you create a window of time for cooking. Begin with every other day. Most of the recipes in this book will make two meals, so you can pack one portion up to eat on the off day. In time, you may go for the ideal of freshly preparing food every day. Foods kept overnight lose a lot of their prana. However, favoring your own cooking over eating out is worth a lot, and relying on leftovers half the time is a great place to start. What Ayurveda doesn't recommend is cooking one pot of food on Sunday and eating it all week long. Once you feel the difference from eating your freshly prepared foods, leftovers will begin to lose their appeal.

> **KITCHEN HINT:** A good time for simmering something is in the morning, while you are getting ready for work and performing your morning routine. You could soak a grain overnight, cook it in a jiffy in the morning, and use half for Creamed Grain Cereal and bring the rest to work to have with soup (instead of bread) or with a Steamed Salad Bowl later.

Let's look at a breakfast example. You probably always get up at a similar time of day and get ready for work. Give yourself half an hour to prepare and sit down to eat one of the template breakfast recipes. Your breakfast is no longer a variable. If you notice that you're sleeping in and compromising your breakfast time, you will know your life is getting out of balance. You are too busy to take care of yourself.

In the appendixes (see page 300), I have provided kitchen techniques for convenience, such as cutting down cooking time by soaking grains and legumes overnight or prechopping some veggies on a day off. This

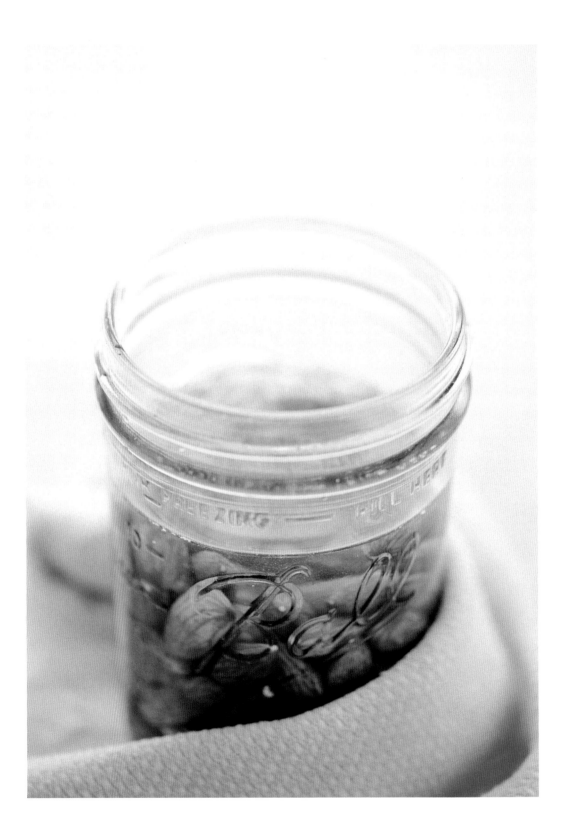

and the simplicity of the recipes, as a rule, are meant to support you in making a positive change.

> If you make a *pattern* of getting up thirty minutes earlier than you're accustomed to, your body will respond by getting sleepy earlier. And if you *listen* to your body, you will move toward an earlier bedtime naturally and consequently enjoy enough rest. Well-digested meals will increase your energy, and you might find you don't need as much sleep as you thought.

Food Combinations

Certain combinations of foods are incompatible, meaning they are likely to ferment in the gut, resulting in gas and bloating, or be too heavy to digest fully, resulting in the creation of ama, the thick, sticky by-product of incomplete digestion. It is considered the substance that begins to cause disease. Think of ama as undigested food that keeps hanging around until it turns into something the body can't easily expel. The following pointers on food combining are good to follow, especially if you aren't feeling well, but remember that an overzealous approach can create stress. One is likely to eat incompatible combinations sometimes, and unless you notice they make you feel bad or you have chronic digestive disorders, relax. If you are making harmonious combinations in your own cooking, your system will be able to process some crazy combinations from time to time. However, if you often feel gassy or bloated after eating, observing correct food combining could turn that around.

MIXING FRUITS WITH OTHER FOODS

Fruit breaks down in the stomach at a faster rate than other foods. When you have fruit and other foods together at the same meal, the stomach will hold the fruit even after it is digested, while it's still breaking down all of the other food. The digested fruit will begin to ferment slightly. Postdigestion, this fermentation will give a sour quality (hot and sharp) to the meal.

Fruits cooked with other foods, however, such as the apples and raisins in Kate's Apple Crisp (see page 229), are less incompatible than raw fruits. Ayurveda teaches that cooking foods together in the pot increases their compatibility by introducing them to each other before they join in the stomach. Recipes never suggest garnishing or making a dessert with uncooked fruits. Eating raw fruit for dessert is not a great habit.

THE DREADED SMOOTHIE: A FOOD-COMBINING NIGHTMARE

The king of incompatible meals is the ice-cold, banana- and milk-based blender bomb known as the smoothie. It seems like a foolproof concept to throw all your nutrition in the carafe with some frozen berries and call it a meal, but on the whole, smoothies are too cold and too complicated for the gut to handle well. This book includes a few warm, fruit-free smoothie recipes for you to check out (see Spiced Nut Milk Smoothie, page 235, and Winter Rejuvenating Tonic, page 279).

If you are an avid smoothie maker, give your gut a break by observing the following guidelines:

- Drink your smoothie at room temperature. Do not make it with ice. If needed, add a few tablespoons of warm water.
- Take cool, fruity smoothies in warm weather only.
- Favor fresh seasonal fruits over frozen.
- Keep the smoothie to three ingredients.
- Do not mix milk and bananas. Both are mucus forming, and together they create too much mucus for the stomach to burn through.
- Add the warming quality of Everyday Sweet Spice Mix (see page 118) to balance a smoothie's cool quality, which can douse digestive fires.

Keep Meals Simple

As a general guideline, keep a meal focused on a major player, like grain or protein, rather than branching out in all directions. Eat enough of the main fare to keep you from grazing afterward. The fewer items you eat in one sitting, the more harmonious your digestion will be. Many of the recipes will suggest a partner dish to help you feel satisfied without your menu getting complicated.

TRY ONE-POT MEALS

Make the one-pot meal a staple of your weekly eating routine. It's easy to make, it travels well, it's filling, and the foods will make a harmonious tune as they cook together. Cooked separately or served raw, these combinations are more difficult to digest. Ayurvedic cookery features a lot of stews, which include spiced combinations of vegetables, lentils and beans, grains and other starches, nuts, and sometimes fruits. I would not recommend eating these foods together in a salad, but cooked together in one pot, it is quite a different story. Remember, it is best not to eat the same meal for several days, so make the right amount of stew for a meal or two, and get in the habit of cooking every day, or at least every other day. The recipes are meant to be quick and simple.

FOODS YOU WILL NOT FIND IN THIS BOOK AND WHY

I've omitted a few foods from the Everyday Ayurveda recipes because of their propensity to promote imbalance. It will generally be OK to have these foods from time to time; however, you will notice they are foods the modern American diet tends to rely on. Learning how to cook without them ensures you are not eating them all the time and gives you a chance to discover if they may be causing you some suffering.

When classifying the qualities of substances, Ayurveda takes into account
- how the qualities of foods are changed by processing
- how the body reacts to foods based on how often the system is accustomed to digesting them

Refined Foods

Eating foods that have been refined into their more subtle aspects—namely, wheat berries refined into flour and sugarcane into bleached, granulated sugar—compounded with the prevalence of these substances in the modern American diet, can provoke imbalance and drain your energy. Ayurveda suggests the prana, or life force, of a food is strongest when the food is as fresh and whole as possible. The digestive tract processes foods best in their original form, and including the natural fibers and minerals of unrefined foods in your diet on a regular basis will ensure your digestive system remains optimal.

Wheat Flour

The intolerance for wheat products, becoming more common all the time, can be due *in some cases* to the refined nature of flour. In refined flour the glutinous, dense, sticky quality of wheat is not accompanied by its natural fibers. This allows the sticky quality to invade the cilia, the tiny hairs inside the small intestine, which are responsible for the wavelike motion of peristalsis, the processing of food through the digestive tract. The sticky quality of flour will disturb the movement of the cilia, and the body will react by producing nausea, gas, and/or diarrhea, telling you not to eat the wheat flour.

Wheat-free flours can ease the problem by replacing the glutinous quality of wheat with dry grains like rice or starch from potato or tapioca. But for Everyday Ayurveda cookery, how about learning some recipes that don't call for flour at all? Dosa, for example, a south Indian flatbread that can stand in for bread or tortillas, is made from soaked and ground rice and legumes. All of the baking recipes in this book will educate you about making baked goods that satisfy the palate and stomach with the use of whole grains, shredded coconut, and nut meals—the ingredients present in traditional Indian sweets. It is OK for most people to have some wheat flour on occasion, but having other options will keep wheat flour from becoming a problem in your diet.

White Sugar

Traditional Ayurveda recommends sugarcane products in varying degrees of refinement, as the cleaning of the pressed sugarcane juice renders it more pure, and a pure form of sweet taste offers building qualities to the body. The modern practice of completely separating sugar from its minerals and bleaching it, however, creates a poisonous food product.

Sugarcane's natural fibers and minerals break down slowly. Separated from its fibers and minerals, the tiny granules of white sugar go too quickly into the bloodstream, causing a spike in the blood sugar. This sudden change in the blood chemistry disturbs the even keel of the entire body, resulting in inconsistent energy levels and a compromised nervous system. With regular use, white sugar can put the body into a constant state of discomfort, contributing to such symptoms as hyperactivity, anxiety, aches and pains, or constipation.

When the Ayurveda classics were codified, more than two thousand years ago, white sugar did not exist as it does now, bleached and isolated from its fibers and minerals. The classic recipes call for jaggery, a dehydrated juice of sugarcane or palm sap. In most stores, you can find evaporated or dehydrated cane juice and coconut sugar. The juice is pressed from the sugarcane or palm fruit and then dried, creating a block that can be broken into granules. Turbinado sugar is dehydrated cane juice that has been spun in a turbine to create large granules and is considered more refined. Less refined sweeteners are preferable to white sugar. And be aware that if a food label lists "sugar" as one of its ingredients, it means white sugar.

Sugarcane itself is not the problem; it is the processing that is problematic. Many other sweet substances in nature are now being rendered into forms to use in daily cooking, such as coconut and date sugars (both quite common in Ayurvedic cookery), maple syrup, and agave. Agave is not featured in this book; however, if it is native to your climate, do seek out the least processed version available and use in the recipes. Honey is revered in Ayurveda, but cooking it is prohibited, as it creates an indigestible, sticky substance the body cannot expel. You will find honey in this book, but not in the baking recipes.

All of these sweet substances have different effects in terms of bringing heating or cooling qualities to the body. Throughout the book they are featured seasonally so you may enjoy the sweet taste, appropriately, in its many forms.

Nightshades

Tomatoes, potatoes, green bell peppers, and eggplant are the nightshade vegetables referenced by Ayurveda. These vegetables contain small amounts of neurotoxins, which may not cause immediate distress but do build in the tissues over time and can result in such symptoms as inflammation of the joints, irritable bowel syndrome, and headaches.

Garlic and Onion

Garlic and onion are foods of medicinal importance. These two offer a pungent taste and a heating quality that are effective in supporting the immune system in cold weather but are too stimulating to be taken regularly as part of the diet. Garlic and onion are known to excite the mind; in some cases this push may be indicated, but generally Ayurveda promotes a peaceful, less reactive nature. To have a small amount of each weekly is probably fine for most people, and yet garlic and onion are everywhere and in everything. Learning how to flavor foods without the use of these hot and bothered standbys is a skill worth having.

Meat

Ayurveda does not require a vegetarian diet. Meat, like all foods, is seen as medicine. Meat would be most appropriate consumed in the cold months or taken in small amounts, cooked into a digestive soup or stew, to build the tissues in conditions of deficiency, recovery from illness, or unwanted weight loss. Classical Ayurveda texts describe the medicinal qualities of different kinds of animal flesh, based on the native climate and activity level of the species. For example, eating beef cultivates cowlike qualities in the body: dense, heavy, slow, static. In Ayurveda, you are what you eat!

The modern Western diet, however, can be dependent on meat, and its consumption often far exceeds medicinal levels. Consider this: the need for the heavy, dense, building qualities of meat on a consistent basis suggests a lifestyle that is taxing the system to the point that it requires the densest of foods in order to keep up. Eating animals is a karma, an action, that binds the body to the more base energies of the universe, called *tamas*, and does not support spiritual energies, *sattva*, as a vegetarian diet does. Take note of whether you are getting enough rest and taking your time to eat fresh, whole foods or whether you are relying on meat to see you through a daily life pattern that is pushing your energetic boundaries. This book provides vegetarian recipes that will nourish you and keep you vital.

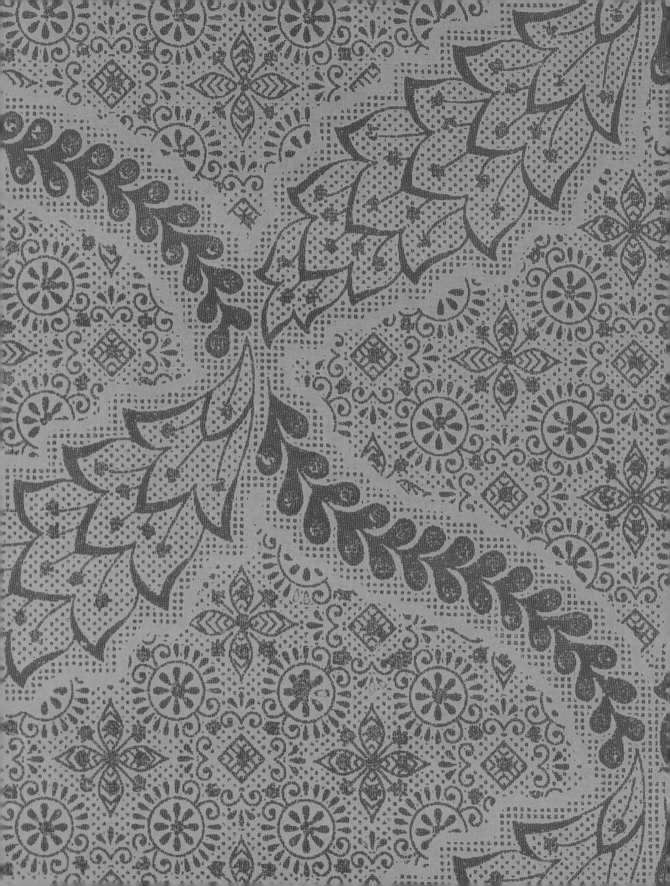

From Theory to Practice

IN THE KITCHEN WITH EVERYDAY AYURVEDA

My yoga teacher, Sri K. Pattabhi Jois, was famous for saying life is "99 percent practice, 1 percent theory." Reading about Ayurveda may help you understand its principles, but it is not until you start experimenting with its diet and lifestyle recommendations that you will begin to see improvements in your health. This chapter is full of tips to help you get your kitchen organized, master the Everyday recipes, and integrate Ayurvedic routines into your daily life. It also provides a road map to what you'll find in part two, "Seasonal Recipes and Routines."

Part two, which follows, features recipes and routines broken out into five chapters of seasonal recipes and lifestyle practices...

Everyday Recipes

DIET: Chapter 5, "Everyday Recipes," contains foundational recipes, beneficial for all bodies, all year long. I have taken great care to offer Everyday recipes that are simple to prepare. Learning how to make these staples is guaranteed to get you started on an Ayurvedic diet. Here you will find the Everyday staples shopping list, which is a great tool to help you start stocking your Ayurvedic pantry and get set up to make the year-round staples.

LIFESTYLE: In addition, in chapter 4 I introduce a few foundational practices that, when gradually worked into a daily routine, will increase immunity, ease aging, and protect the body/mind from stress.

Spring, Summer, Fall, Winter

Each of the four seasonal chapters begins with a review of the elements and qualities most prevalent in that season, as well as the signs and symptoms of imbalance to watch for.

DIET: In each chapter I introduce the qualities and tastes for encouraging balance during that season, as well as including a table showing what foods to favor. These foods are then organized into a season-specific shopping list, ensuring you will have on hand whatever you need to make the recipes featured in that chapter.

LIFESTYLE: To encourage optimal health through the changing season, in each chapter I expand the basic daily routine with a few key actions.

Chapter 3 Helps You . . .

GET ORGANIZED
- Balancing Everyday recipes and seasonal recipes
- Organizing the Everyday pantry and spice rack
- Using the seasonal shopping lists

GET INTUITIVE: WHEN AND HOW TO MODIFY THE RECIPES
- Adapting for different climates
- Cooking for the family
- Adapting for travel
- Integrating *dinacharya* (lifestyle practices)

Think of Ayurveda as a hobby. Integrating new ways of taking care of yourself (for example, cooking the majority of your own food) can take awhile. If you were to take up the hobby of knitting, you would benefit by first buying a skein or two of yarn and learning how to make something simple. Otherwise it would be easy to end up with a basket full of yarns, a head full of design ideas, and very little staying power. Once you settle in and feel the simplicity of what Ayurveda is teaching, you can chuckle at what a big deal it may have seemed to get started. Simply begin by getting a few of the Everyday recipes under your belt. Remember, it helps to turn your attention to making new habits with an eye toward exploration, self-acceptance, and sense of humor.

Finding a Flow with Everyday Recipes

The Everyday recipes suggest a three-meal-a-day flow for eating food you have prepared, all year round—ideally, a medium-size breakfast to suit your appetite, a big lunch, and a small supper. The suggested seasonal mix-ins provide some variety, but the cooking method doesn't change from season to season, so you are not reinventing the wheel every time the weather shifts. Think of the Everyday recipes as templates. Once you get the hang of the basics, you can get more creative with what vegetables, oils, or spices you are using to make an Everyday dish. To help you along, I've included a number of seasonal recipes that use an Everyday recipe as a template.

If you don't get bored easily, you could eat solely from the Everyday recipes and enjoy an affordable, unprocessed, manageable diet rich in qualities that promote balance. When you are ready, expand your Everyday fare by branching out into the recipes in the seasonal chapters, and I hope you will find soon enough that you don't need a recipe anymore to whip up something satisfying.

KEEP IT SIMPLE: Remember, especially when you start playing with mix-ins, that the efficacy of Ayurvedic cookery is in its simplicity. Allow your tastes to gradually favor meals that contain few ingredients. Eat a hearty portion of one dish, rather than a smorgasbord of small bites. Keep it simple and you'll feel better.

FROM THEORY TO PRACTICE

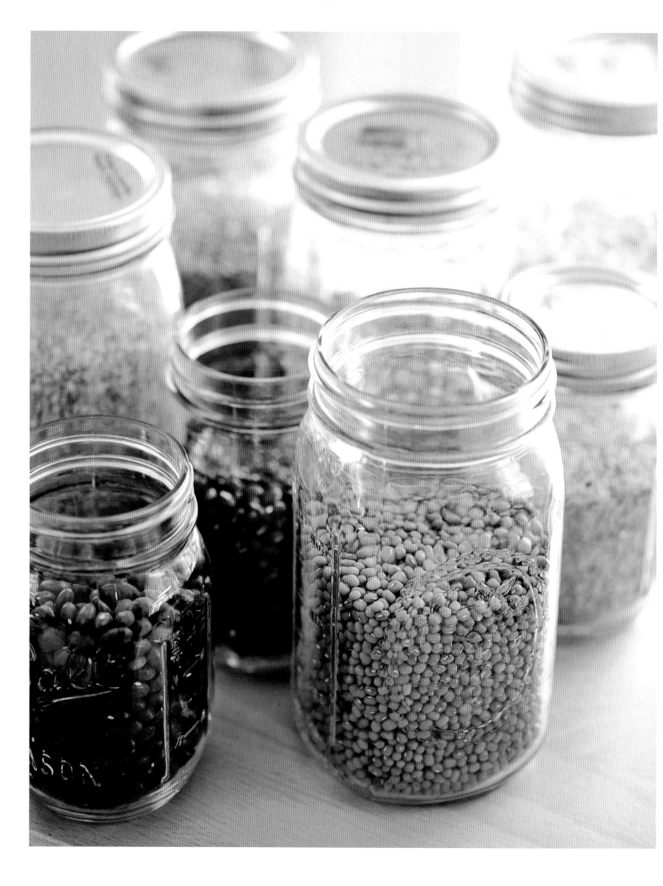

Creating a diet that changes with the seasons is a lifestyle practice anchored in awareness of how your body feels. The recipes in this book suggest food ideas that will ease the transitions, but it's your job to pay attention to the changing qualities of the months. With practice and a few seasons behind you, your intuition and creativity to change your diet year-round will become second nature. Keep it fun and flexible.

Organizing the Everyday Pantry and Spice Rack

Store your staple grains, legumes, nuts, and dried fruits in glass jars. Using glass jars for storage keeps the pantry neat and pretty to look at. To avoid having miscellaneous plastic bags peeking out from behind each other on your shelves or gathering in piles only to be forgotten, you'll find it worthwhile to take the time to procure some nice-looking jars that will fit together on a shelf or in a drawer. In any case it's a good idea to move away from using plastics for kitchen storage, as they are all made from chemicals, and you can't be sure if these are leeching into your foods over time. You can use canning jars, which come in several sizes and have two-part metal tops for easy cleaning and storage. These can be found at hardware and kitchen/home supply stores.

TIFFIN, INDIAN LUNCH BOX

The word *tiffin* can refer to a small meal or to the container small meals are packed in. In most parts of India, food is stored in stainless steel containers with latching tops, sometimes stackable for holding separate dishes of rice, dal, and vegetables. It is common to see locals riding bicycles to work with three-tiered lunch tiffins swinging from their handlebars. Tiffins are available at Indian markets and natural foods stores in a variety of shapes and sizes.

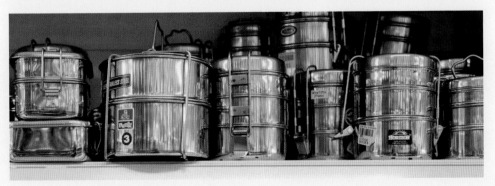

Canning jars for storage, 16-ounce and 32-ounce sizes

Leakproof glass food storage containers in a variety of sizes

Insulated lunch bag (if you often eat away from home); look for a waterproof one that fits neatly into your work tote.

Glass or steel water bottle (for warm weather)

Drink thermos (to replace water bottle in cool weather); look for stainless steel and leakproof.

Soup thermos, stainless steel and with a wide mouth for hot meals on the go

Pepper mill

3-ounce glass jars with shaker tops (for Ayurvedic spice mixes and salts)

Mortar and pestle (for grinding spices)

HERBS AND SPICES

You'll enjoy the optimal medicinal value of spices by buying them whole, which are good for about one year, and grinding up a batch monthly. Once a seed has been ground up, its flavor and efficacy will diminish after about a month.

Traditional Ayurvedic cookery often calls for both whole spices and ground spices in a soup, stew, rice, or cooked vegetable recipe. The body of the dish will be flavorful from the powdered spices, while the whole seeds add bursts of extra flavor and visual variety. In the recipes in this book, the whole spices are sometimes optional. When you're starting out, it's best to grind up a batch of seasoning monthly—meeting all your needs for taste, seasonal qualities, and good digestion—and just use that. As you get more discerning with your cookery, you may start to augment the recipes with whole spices as well, for variety and excitement.

Buy spices at a natural foods store that carries bulk culinary herbs and spices, or you can order them from an Ayurvedic supply company (see "Resources," page 320). One-half pound of each type of spice is a good amount to order.

Storage. Keep your spices in glass jars or, if you are lucky enough to find one, in a spice box (see page 59), the traditional way of storing Indian spices; the flavors meld into a masala inside the box. Pint-sized jars hold a good amount of whole spices to keep around, to be used within one year. Saving and washing glass nut-butter jars from the grocery store is a thrifty way to gather a uniform collection; another option is to purchase canning jars.

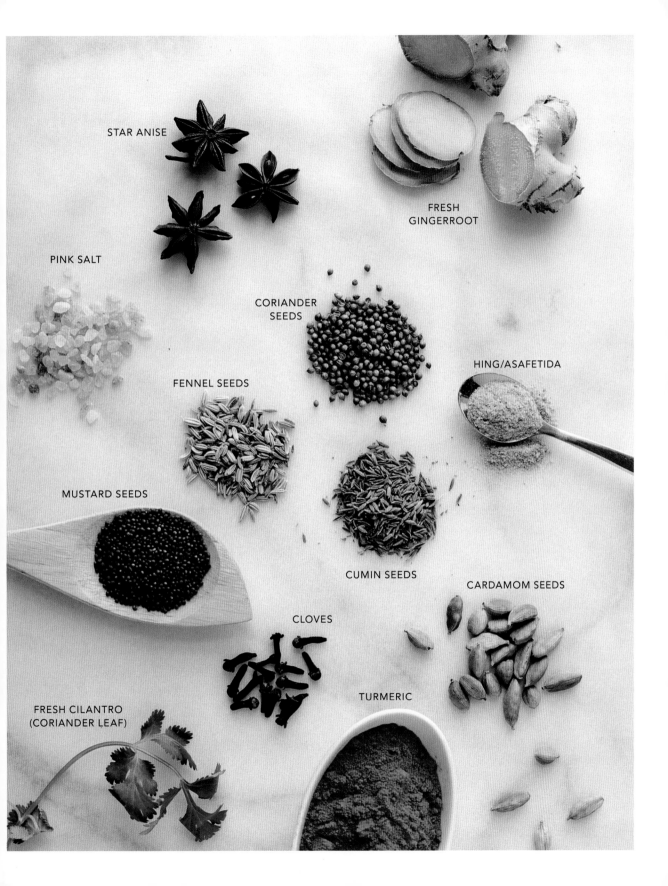

STAR ANISE

FRESH GINGERROOT

PINK SALT

CORIANDER SEEDS

HING/ASAFETIDA

FENNEL SEEDS

MUSTARD SEEDS

CUMIN SEEDS

CARDAMOM SEEDS

CLOVES

FRESH CILANTRO
(CORIANDER LEAF)

TURMERIC

For daily use, in the spice rack or on the back of the stove, keep ground spices in a few small glass jars with shaker tops, which can also be found at any kitchen or home goods store. Have a pepper mill filled with fresh peppercorns on the table.

To make the Everyday spice mixes you will need:

- Coriander seed
- Fennel seed
- Cumin seed

The following spices are best bought in powdered form, as they are difficult to grind up on your own:

- Turmeric
- Cardamon (though whole green pods are beautiful in rice dishes and chai)
- Cinnamon
- Ginger
- Pink salt or sea salt

Once you get in the habit of using the seasonal shopping lists, you will buy a few extra spices each season and can vary the mixtures in your shaker jars, making one just for Ayurvedic tastes and another for the Western-style recipes.

Fresh herbs are always best, but they are not always easy to find. All year round, you can grow a few culinary favorites in pots on your windowsill and cut bits for fresh garnishes. Parsley, thyme, rosemary, and mint all grow pretty well inside.

When herbs are fresh in season, you can buy them at the farmers' market and hang them up in bunches to dry in your kitchen, then store in glass jars. These can be used to make the seasonal salts. Dried culinary herbs can also be purchased at a natural foods store that carries bulk spices. A little goes a long way, so just buy a quarter cup or so for the season. If you are cooking for a family, buy closer to one-half cup.

FRESH GINGER

Fresh gingerroot is paramount and should be purchased weekly and kept outside the refrigerator. Look for roots with small fingers, which will be tender and delicate in flavor. In the latter part of the harvest season, you will find "young ginger" at the farmers' market. These roots are small, pink, and appear medicinally in classic Ayurvedic cookery. Buy them and use them as much as you can when they are around.

Also known as a masala box, this stainless steel circular canister is a traditional way of storing Ayurvedic spices. The canister holds a number of small cups for individual spices, both whole and ground, which are then allowed to harmonize their flavors inside the box. Cooks can access the full spice cabinet by pulling out only one container. I love my spice box tremendously, and it holds seven cups: turmeric powder, coriander powder, peppercorns, cumin seed, coriander seed, fennel seed, and mustard seed. I also have a separate box for sweet-tasting chai spices. As you discover your favorite flavors from the lists here, pick the seven MVPs and feature them in your very own spice box.

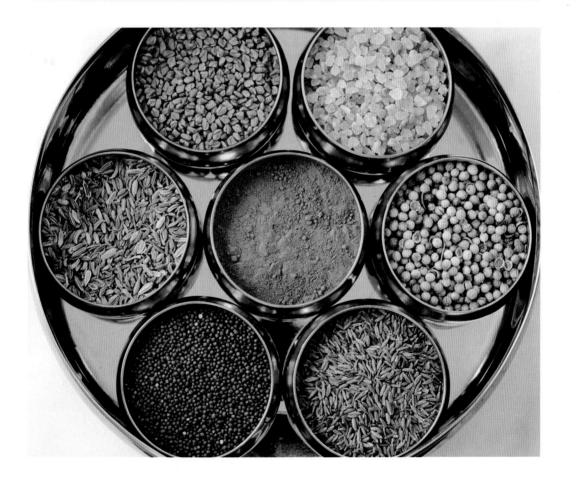

GRAINS AND LEGUMES

Have fun varying your grains and legumes with the seasonal shopping lists, but keep a few superstars in quart-sized jars for the Everyday recipes. When cooking for a family, you may store larger bags in the pantry, if you find a quart jar goes too fast to keep refilling.

- Basmati rice, brown and white
- Mung beans, whole green and split yellow

NUTS, SEEDS, AND DRIED FRUITS

Seeds are lighter than nuts and appear in recipes throughout all four seasons, while nuts come and go on your seasonal lists. Dried fruits are favored on a seasonal basis and appear mostly when fresh fruits are not available, so just stock them seasonally. Store the following in glass jars in the refrigerator:

- Raw sunflower seeds
- Raw almonds
- Shredded coconut
- Chia seeds

GREAT DATES

Dried dates, usually of the deglet noor variety, are free of pits and convenient for baking. However, Ayurveda tells us "wet" dates are preferable to dried, because they are fresh (more prana) and easier on the blood sugar. If you can get fresh dates, buy them as you would any fruit, but in cooler climates, buy the Medjool date, which is as close to fresh as you will find. If you don't mind removing the pits, use these instead of dried when you can.

OILS

Consuming fresh oils is important. Oils go rancid, and the body cannot metabolize them in this form, which results in ama, undigested toxic matter in the tissues. You do not want to have cooking oils around more than a few months. The seasonal shopping lists will guide you to buy seasonally appropriate oils so you can use them up, then shift into the next season's variety. For example, some oils, like sesame, are heavier than others and therefore more appropriate in cool weather; coconut oil has a cooling quality and so is recommended in warm weather. However, Everyday Ghee (see page 120) is beneficial all year long and keeps well for one month outside of the refrigerator and up to three months in the fridge.

Remember: ghee and coconut oil have the greatest heat tolerance (they don't turn rancid at high heat) and are used in all the baked goods recipes in this book. Other cooking oils, such as olive and sesame, can tolerate medium heat and are acceptable for stove-top cooking.

Using the Seasonal Shopping Lists

Celebrate the changes in seasons by spending a little time "seasonalizing" your pantry, in the same way you change out your seasonal clothing. Rather than keeping only the same oils, grains, nuts, dried fruits, and legumes stocked all year long, get excited about the foods and flavors you haven't seen for a while. Taking the time to appreciate the variety nature gives us will feed your soul and your senses.

Each recipe chapter contains a seasonal shopping list designed to guide you into buying foods that will balance the qualities changing in your body at that time of year and that will keep your diet pleasantly varied. When you use the list for stocking up, you will be prepared to make most of the recipes for the season.

As the qualities in your environment begin to shift, phase out the foods that do not appear on the new season's list by using up what you have. Take a few hours to prepare or purchase items from the new season's shopping list, then return home to get things organized in the kitchen. Change out what's in your glass jars; the varieties of legumes, grains, nuts, and oils you are stocking; and make up some fresh, seasonally appropriate spice and salt mixes. You are then ready to make the recipes featured in the new season's chapter and to balance the qualities in your body by gently attending to your diet.

You will find many suggested fresh fruits and vegetables on the shopping lists. Don't buy them all at once! Only buy enough fresh fruit and vegetables for one week's meals at a time. Buy just a couple varieties of fruit and veggie in one trip considering how many you are cooking for. Buy more vegetables than fruits. To keep it simple, try rotating the fruits and veggies you buy each time you go shopping so that you can try all the varieties. Buy only as much as you can prepare and eat in a few days or a workweek, to ensure you keep eating fresh produce and avoid spoilage. As a rule, if something looks great to you, your body probably wants to eat it. (We are not talking about brownies here.) Buy a new vegetable that attracts you and try it in one of the recipes. Each time you experiment with unfamiliar produce, you expand your cookery skills.

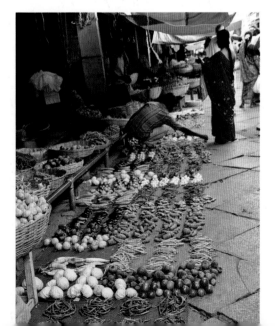

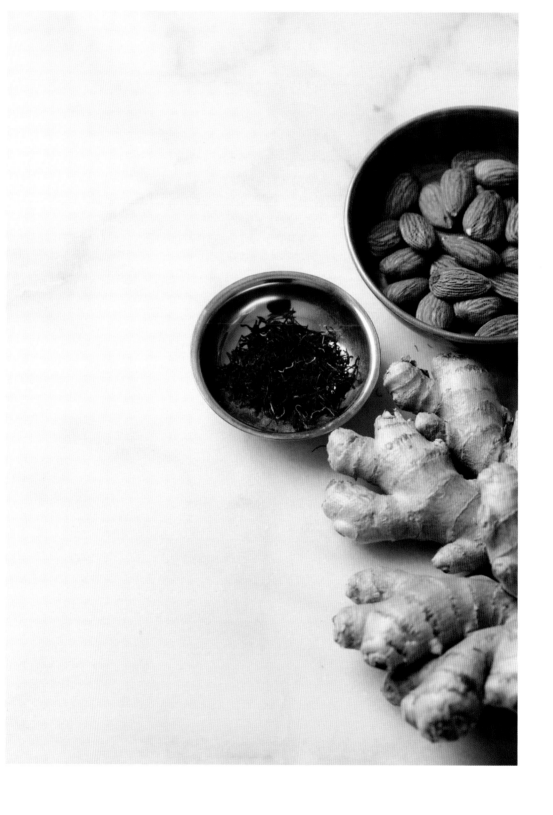

Remember, the Everyday recipes are meant to guide you to prepare meals simply from the staple ingredients you keep around all the time. If you don't get around to rotating the pantry right away when the season changes, it's OK—just keep cooking!

Recipe Yields

The more complicated a recipe is, the larger the recipe yield. The logic of this is simple: If you are putting a lot of time into cooking a dish, you likely want to have more of the final product to enjoy. Most of *The Everyday Ayurveda Cookbook* recipes are uncomplicated and will yield two servings, whereas soups and stews that need to simmer awhile generally serve four. (Note: This could be four demure bowls, if the soup is a side dish, or two big bowls, if the soup is your main meal.) Rather than teaching you to get fancy in the kitchen, make large amounts of food, and eat leftovers often, *The Everyday Ayurveda Cookbook* seeks to get you cooking more simply and more often. More fresh foods equal more vibrant health.

Some of you will be cooking for yourselves alone and will eat half of a dish at one sitting and keep half to use for the next meal or to take to work. If you are cooking for two, double the recipe so both people can benefit from a packed lunch tomorrow.

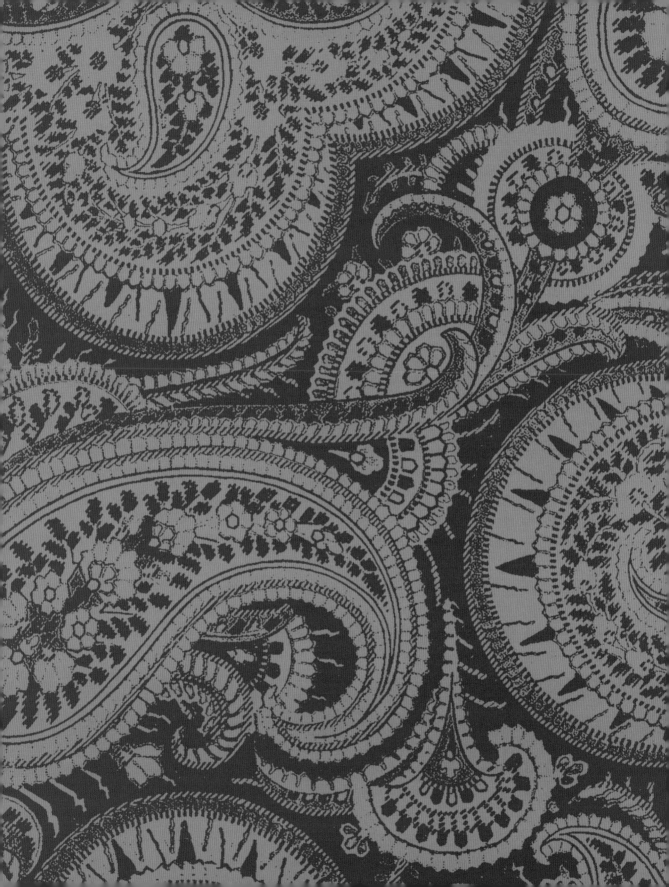

CHAPTER 4

Adapting for Your Life

CLIMATE, FAMILY, AND TRAVEL

Throughout my twenty-five plus years of introducing people to the principles of Ayurvedic eating, the top three questions I hear are always the same:

> *What if I don't have seasons like the four outlined in* The Everyday Ayurveda Cookbook?
>
> *What if my family members each need different qualities in their foods—am I supposed to cook different dishes for everyone?*
>
> *What about when I travel?*

If you are wondering any of the above, you are in good company. Fear not, the Everyday Ayurveda principles are meant to be adapted to support your life. Adapting Ayurveda's knowledge of balancing the qualities of body, environment, and food works anywhere you are, with whomever you find yourself.

Read on to discover how to adapt the seasonal qualities to your home place, as well as accounting for the climate *inside* your body. Here you will also find strategies for the family cook (don't worry—you do not need to cook different dishes for everyone!) and my tried-and-true travel hacks to keep the Ayurveda lifestyle moving with you through life.

Cooking for the Family

If you are cooking to feed a family, you will want to double or triple most of the recipes. However, one of the joys of this book is that it shows you how simple it is to cook something just for yourself. Your body might not be calling for the meat and potatoes or mac 'n' cheese that is typical American family fare. Instead, you might parboil some fresh greens, use an immersion hand blender to process half into a simple green soup for you (Everyday Cleansing Green Soup, page 108), and serve the other half of the parboiled vegetables as a side dish for the rest of the crowd. You can augment your soup with a little meat and eat much less potato than you would have without your side soup. Teaching you to stay true to what you need, without feeling over-whelmed by cooking several meals at once, is one of the aims of this book.

To personalize the Everyday template recipes, family members can choose their own mix-ins to add to each basic meal. At breakfast, for instance, serve a batch of Everyday Creamed Grain Cereal (page 84) cooked with slightly less water than the recipe calls for and offer, as an addition, cow's milk for one person and almond milk for another. Or serve Everyday Steamed Salad Bowl (page 94) for dinner, but offer two or three of the dressing choices and several different toppings on the side—one person can have meat, another can have toasted seeds.

Notes for the Family Chef:

- Keeping spice mixes handy in shaker jars invites each eater to spice the meal according to his or her tastes.
- Keep a jar of ghee or coconut oil available, along with a clean spoon, for those who need to add more oil to a meal.
- Most Indian households have a pressure cooker. If you are willing to learn how to use one, this is a speedy way to produce butter-soft beans and vegetables. According to Ayurvedic cooking, pressure cooking is the best way to ensure digestibility of dry, hard foods. Slow cooking is another method that requires more planning but softens foods nicely as well.
- Kids need sweet taste, and naturally sweetened cooking will build taste buds that don't demand white sugar. Dates or raisins cooked in Everyday Kichari (page 100) are sure to go "down the hatch" easily, as my dad used to say.
- Make up new batches of chutneys, sauces, and spreadables every week. If someone at the table doesn't instantly love the meal you've served, maybe she or he will love it with mango chutney on top.
- Kids are in the building phase of life and so need more of the heavy, dense foods, like dairy products, eggs, sweet potatoes, and nut butters.

The muffin recipes in this book could be a lifesaver for you, the family chef, and are good in the lunchbox. Don't tell them what it's called, but Winter Rejuvenating Tonic (see page 279) is also ideally nourishing for children and grounds their energy after a school day.

• Growing children generally need to eat more often and to consume less at each meal than adults. But even if you feed your children five times a day, try to stick to eating three meals yourself.

Adapting for Different Climates

Take a moment to review the table "The Ten Builders and Their Opposites" (see page 14). It is important to feel for these qualities as you notice your daily sensations and watch for any early symptoms of imbalance. Once you understand how the recipes are using foods to balance the seasonal qualities, you can modify the recipes to balance the qualities at work in your own body. When in doubt, reach for the neutral foods suggested in the Everyday recipes.

The following qualities form the basis for the seasonal recipe chapters.

SPRING: heavy, oily/damp, slow, cloudy, stable

SUMMER: hot, sharp/bright, oily/humid

FALL: cool, light, dry, rough, mobile (windy), clear

WINTER: cool, very dry, light, rough, mobile, hard, clear

YOUR INDOOR ENVIRONMENT

Remember, if you spend a lot of time indoors, you will need to account for the environment inside, which may be the same all year long. Both air-conditioning and heat are dry, dry, dry. Some workplaces, like office buildings and retail shops, may be kept very cold, so adjust for that when planning food and drink for your workdays.

Spring foods are drying and warming, as they are meant to melt winter residue, and they call for very little salt. If spring in your area is generally less damp and cool than a typical spring environment, you can enjoy a bit more salt and a bit more oil in the recipes.

Summer foods will be light on the oil and cooling in nature. If your summer is dry instead of humid, you can add more fats and oils to the recipes.

Fall recipes favor warm, cooked foods, though without any ingredients that are *too* heating, like chilies. The foods will be building, grounding, well oiled, and deeply nourishing to prepare the body for a long winter. If the winter you expect is not so long as in a cold environment, consume building foods for a shorter period. With a longer growing season, you will also enjoy adding more fresh vegetables to the recipes.

Winter recipes favor slightly heating foods, served warm, watery, and oily, with a bit of spice. If your winter is not very dry and cold—for instance, if you live in a climate where it rains all winter—you may favor the winter recipes for their warming effects, but cut back a bit on the oils and heavy fats. In this case, reduce the sour, salty tastes as well, as they cause the body to hold water.

Understanding Internal Climate

In actuality, you have two climates to consider when making your food choices: that of your external environment and, more important, your internal climate. Each body contains a unique makeup of the five Ayurvedic elements. It is possible, for example, to be born with a propensity to be cold and dry, even during seasons that present warm and moist qualities.

A cold individual might feel the strongest and most integrated during the warm months and can relax a bit on keeping warm and oiled at this time, but this individual certainly *doesn't* need to seek out cooling, drying foods at any time of year. He is likely to experience cold hands and feet most of the time. He *can* get away with having some favorite cool and dry foods more often in the warm weather, should the mood move him. Eating too much from the spring recipes is likely to make this person uncomfortable and perhaps cause dry skin or gassiness. Simply by adding some good fats and oils to his meals, he will experience relief.

Another person might experience a hot internal environment, which could manifest as acid stomach or a feeling of toastiness, even in winter. Perhaps the internal heat is worse in summer. She would do well to reduce the intake of such sharp items as coffee and alcohol. Instead, focus on summer drinkables and enjoy cooling condiments, such as Cilantro Mint Chutney, all year round.

Yet another individual gains weight easily all year long, particularly in winter. Although it is light and dry outside in winter, this body holds heavy and oily qualities inside. The winter diet may prove too rich for him. Favoring some of the drying, astringent grains and vegetables from the spring chapter will help make some of the winter recipes lighter for this person.

The truth is that eating simply and noticing how different foods make you feel or what qualities they present (Comfortably warm? Aggravated? Heavy after eating, or energized?) informs your understanding of how to modify the recipes for your internal climate.

Some Don't Like It Hot

Cindy's least favorite weather is that of a steamy summer day. Her rosy complexion turns bright red when she gets hot, she has a tendency toward burping, and she often gets acid indigestion from spicy food. Cindy also notices she is prone to acne before her menstrual cycle, especially when she has that second iced coffee in the afternoon every day and indulges in the habit of postwork cocktails. When things get stressful at the office, sometimes she has to run for the toilet right after meals. Not surprisingly, winter is her favorite time of year, and the cold weather makes her feel energized.

Cindy's natural preference for winter and her tendencies toward overheating, acid stomach, acne, and quick digestion all suggest a hot internal environment. She is likely to notice these tendencies fire up in humid weather, when sharp, oily, heating qualities predominate. Eating recipes from the summer chapter will ease the symptoms of internal heat at any time of year. Cindy might enjoy a bit of spicy food on occasion in the cold weather, but she knows better than to go for it when it is hot outside. She is fond of having Cardamom Limeade and Cilantro Mint Chutney with her meals all year round. She loves coffee, but she can tell when she is drinking too much of it—her stomach tends to be more acidic, and she gets hungry—so avoids having it on an empty stomach.

Sticky Stuff

Frank is always trying to lose a little weight. It seems like if he has a piece of pastry (which he is always craving, especially when he isn't on his exercise regimen), he can't burn it off. Once he gets started exercising, he has great stamina, but if he doesn't get to it in the morning, he will feel sluggish and unmotivated all day. His skin is often clammy and cool to the touch, though he wouldn't tell you he feels cold. His least favorite time of year is spring, when he is often congested and can't taste anything. Warm, dry weather makes Frank feel lighter and more apt to go outside.

Frank's natural aversion to damp weather and his tendencies toward weight gain and congestion suggest a damp, cool internal environment. Though it seems to come to a head in late winter or spring, for him congestion can result from eating a big dinner or an ice cream cone at any time of the year. If Frank chooses light, dry recipes from the spring chapter whenever he feels sluggish or congested, he can alleviate these symptoms of a damp internal environment. He really likes the autumnal Cranberry Butternut Muffin recipe all year round, but he has learned to go for the spring recipes of Savory Breakfast Soup or Berry Buck-Up Cereal if it's a rainy, cold day, or else he feels heavy all morning.

A Big Chill

Phyllis is always cold; she can't go anywhere without a sweater in her bag. If she drinks iced water at a restaurant and has only a salad, she will have trouble getting warm again. She might order hot soup even when it's warm out—but not with beans, because they give her gas. She always has a hard time in winter, gets very dry skin, and isn't likely to eliminate daily. Phyllis is happiest in a warm bath or on vacation in the tropics.

Phyllis's love for warm bathing and hot soup suggests a cold internal environment. She is likely to feel better eating fall and winter recipes most of the time. The grounding, moist qualities of these foods will help her stay warm and comfortable. She knows to wait for hot weather before enjoying a salad, and even then, she takes care to eat cooked food more often than raw, because she finds she has less gas and bloating this way.

Use the "Seasonal Signs and Symptoms" table often to review the signs and symptoms of imbalance and the qualities at work in each case. (See also "Recipe Index by Symptoms" in appendix 4.) This will help you to recognize what qualities are in need of balance and whether they correspond to the season at hand or are present only in your body.

SEASONAL SIGNS AND SYMPTOMS		
SEASON	QUALITIES OF THE SEASON	SIGNS AND SYMPTOMS OF IMBALANCE
SPRING	Cool, heavy, oily (damp), slow, cloudy, stable	Congestion, seasonal allergies, weight gain, water retention, lethargy, sadness
SUMMER	Hot, sharp (bright), oily (humid)	Acid indigestion, reflux, loose stools, pimples, rashes, swelling, irritability, headaches
FALL	Cool, light, dry, rough, mobile (windy), clear, erratic, early fall is also hot	Gas and bloating, constipation, dry skin and scalp, itchy or burning rashes, cold hands and feet, insomnia, anxiety
WINTER	Cold, very dry, light, rough, mobile, hard, clear	Constipation, dry skin and scalp, cracking joints, cold hands and feet, anxiety, fatigue

The prevalence of sound and light (even at night), billboards and other advertisements, the vibration of electronics, the movement of vehicles—all of these elements of urban environs increase the mobile quality of the mind and the activity of the sense organs. Both of these effects require some balancing. Regardless of the season, city dwellers need to nurture stable, dense, slow, and soft qualities. For example, meditation, oil massage, or gentle yoga will help cultivate these qualities, as will seeking out contact with the natural world (grass, leaves, flowers, even a pet) and taking a few moments to feel the soft quality on the skin.

Taking It on the Road: Travel Tips

If you travel away from home to a different climate, you will notice in a day or two how the qualities of the new environment affect you. If you are suddenly surrounded by humidity and you aren't used to that, it will feel especially moist and warm to you, and you will crave dry and cooling qualities. Be prepared to change your diet while you are in this new place, the same way you would for a changing season. Also, be aware that the qualities of air travel are incredibly dry and light. If you're flying, make it a point to eat warm, moist food and oil your skin upon arrival–these simple practices will balance the effects of air travel.

You needn't lose your Everyday Ayurveda routine when you travel. Again, the key is to be prepared. You'll run into trouble when traveling when you don't have any oil for oil massage, when you forgot your thermos. Keeping a travel kit ready in a clear plastic bag for flights will help you maintain your routine while you're on the road. It should include:

- A tongue scraper (see page 288)
- A three-ounce, leakproof plastic bottle of massage oil. Before your flight be sure to put some of the oil inside your nose, inhaling deeply. Or purchase a *nasya* oil for your travel kit (see page 291). A shower and oil massage (*abhyanga*) after you land will do wonders to balance the drying effects of flying (see page 292).
- Rose water hydrosol. If your eyes get dry, spray or drop rose water into them.
- Ginger tea bags. Do not have iced drinks or alcohol on the plane; ask for hot water for tea.
- Triphala, if you tend to get constipated (see sidebar)

Triphala (pronounced "tri-fuh-la") means "three fruits." It is a mild, cleansing formula made by compounding three dried fruits: *amalaki*, *haritaki*, and *bibhitaki*. Available at most health food stores, triphala is great for establishing regularity during travel and times of stress. This compound repairs and soothes the organs of digestion and elimination, and it contains five of the six tastes. Triphala is generally appropriate for most body types. Consult an Ayurvedic practitioner for dosage and usage.

Pack a thermos or glass or steel water bottle. If you're flying, ask the flight attendant for warm water in your bottle.

Sometimes it's hard to find unprocessed foods when you're traveling. The good news is that an Ayurvedic diet at home improves your digestive capacity, so if you end up having to eat at a diner once in a while, your digestive fire will get right to work. But if you find yourself eating processed foods every night of your trip, you could end up experiencing signs of imbalance, such as bloating, gas, acid stomach, or irregularity. When eating out at restaurants, request hot water with lemon or mint tea to drink; focus on eating grain dishes and roasted and steamed vegetables; and ask for real olive oil and lemon wedges or balsamic vinegar to dress your salads. Remember, you have a choice about what you put into your body, even at a restaurant, and if you ask for vegetables, the kitchen will always come up with something.

Now Is the Time

Integrating the Ayurvedic diet, lifestyle practices, and wisdom into your life may take some time. It is most enjoyable—and effective—to start with something simple, and remember that small changes are lasting ones.

So, friends, let's get cooking. Turn the page and begin to change your life, one meal at a time.

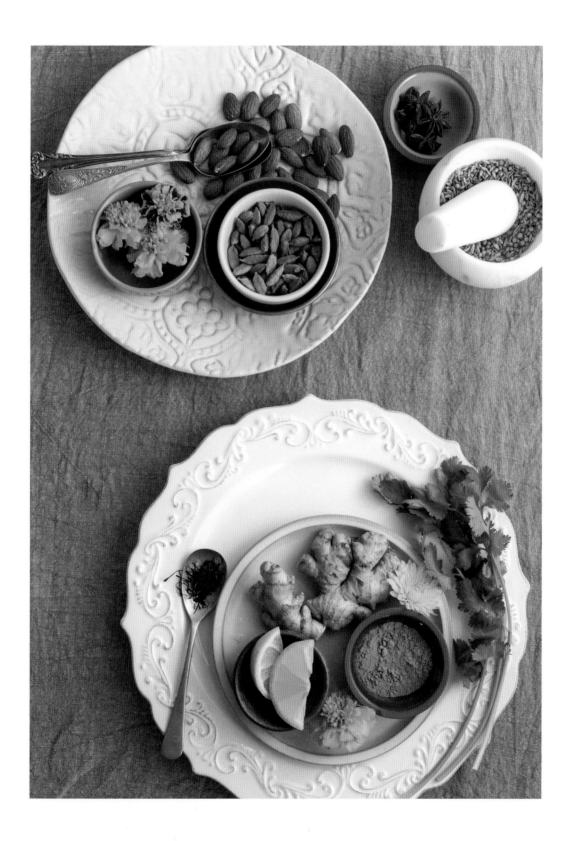

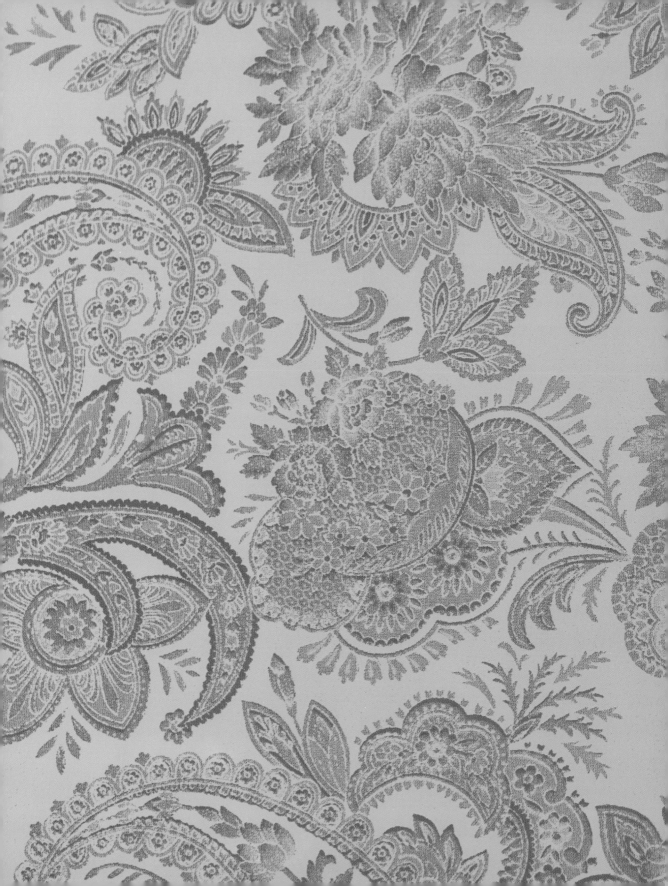

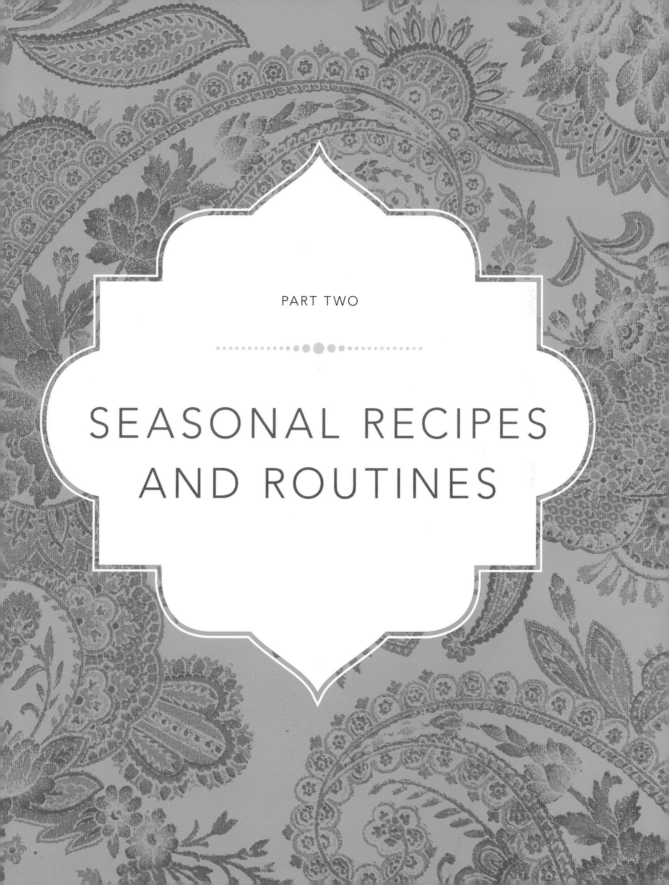

PART TWO

SEASONAL RECIPES AND ROUTINES

CHAPTER 5

Everyday Recipes

FOUNDATIONAL DISHES
FOR YEAR-ROUND COOKING

To get started in your Ayurvedic kitchen, this chapter provides a basic and balanced selection of recipes that are appropriate all year. They will help you maintain a state of wellness, supported by your own cooking. The Everyday recipes are complete foundations, and they can be varied by optional mix-ins to accommodate the changing qualities in your seasonal atmosphere and appetite. If you start by mastering these basic, versatile recipes, you will be well on the way to eating more of your own cooking and to learning how to be creative, quick, and satisfied in the kitchen. Moreover, you will notice improvements in your health and the quality of your digestion.

What makes an Everyday recipe?

- The Everyday recipes are neutral (as opposed to cooling or heating), are served warm, and are made only with whole foods.
- None of these recipes contains a lengthy list of ingredients or takes a long time to prepare.

Each of these dishes is important enough in Ayurvedic cookery—or just so darn convenient—that it's worth taking the time to learn how to make them all.

What Is a Mix-in?

A mix-in is an optional food addition to your meal that will bring one or more of the six tastes, and their beneficial qualities, to your food. In most cases, the Everyday recipes are basic and neutral in taste. Mix-ins give you the opportunity to rotate different foods and tastes in a seasonal rhythm. For example, Everyday Creamed Grain Cereal is very simple and provides the building, grounding qualities of sweet taste, as does any grain dish. In damp weather, however, you could add the dry quality of astringent taste by mixing in raisins. In cold weather, you could increase the moist, dense qualities by adding dates and a teaspoon of ghee, balancing the density with a blast of pungent ginger powder. Used this way, the Everyday recipes become your baseline, and because they are versatile, you won't get bored with your cooking.

On another note, mix-ins can spruce up a simple dish without creating indigestible food combinations. For example, if a bowl of oatmeal for breakfast doesn't provide enough fuel for you to make it to lunch without snacking, you might need to add a little something extra, such as some nuts or a poached egg (but not both). Choose from the mix-ins listed for each season, and note when the directions say to use A *or* B (to avoid using both in the same meal). Simple meals will sustain you longer yet still digest well, providing clean-burning fuel straight through to the next meal.

Everyday Food Guide

FOODS TO FAVOR YEAR-ROUND

- Neutral foods and spices; cooked grains, legumes, and vegetables.
- Most meals served warm.
- Green vegetables in season: if it's green and it's in season, eat it. Kale and collards can be harvested even during the winter in some areas.

- Neutral fruits, fresh and ripe, such as apples and pears (cooked in cold weather).
- Mung beans and white basmati rice, the most digestible bean and easy grain combination for any season.
- Sunflower, chia, hemp, sesame, and flaxseeds.
- Ghee and coconut oil for cooking and baking.
- Moderate amounts of neutral spices, such as parsley, coriander, cumin, fennel, cinnamon, cardamom, gingerroot, and turmeric.
- Sea vegetables, such as kombu and dulse.
- Fresh homemade almond milk and soaked almonds.
- Fresh yogurt, diluted with water (lassi).

FOODS TO REDUCE YEAR-ROUND
- Caffeine, especially coffee (and any coffee you drink should be organic).
- White sugar.
- Alcoholic beverages.
- Nightshades: raw tomatoes; eggplant; bell peppers, especially green; white potatoes.
- Garlic and onion (limit to once or twice a week).
- Cold food and drink.
- Fermented foods, especially store-bought or old: pickled fruits and vegetables, kombucha, aged cheeses, and kimchi. Use sparingly, as condiments.

General Year-Round Lifestyle Guidelines

The following dinacharya routines may take a little time to incorporate into your life, and you don't have to make all these changes right away. As you try them, one by one, watch how these new habits increase your vibrance and productivity in your daily life. You will find that some of these habits are more important for you than others, and it's more helpful to stick with these few than trying to do it all.

- Scrape your tongue first thing in the morning, before drinking or eating anything (see page 288).
- Rinse the eyes a few times with cool water (see page 290).
- Instead of making a beeline for the coffeepot, begin the day with the Easy Morning Beverage (see page 110), which takes just as little if not less time than brewing coffee or caffeinated tea.

- Oil the skin daily with neutral oils, such as almond, sunflower, or safflower (see page 292).
- Get to bed by 10 P.M. and wake up naturally with the sun.
- Reduce screen time (TV, smartphone, computer) upon waking and after 9 P.M.
- Exercise moderately, most days, for thirty to forty-five minutes. Exercise just to the point when sweat begins to form, then cool down.
- Walk outside in fresh air every day.
- Avoid drinking water one-half hour before meals and wait at least one hour after eating to drink more water.
- Drink six ounces of ginger, tulsi, or fennel tea with or after meals.
- Eat only when hungry; reduce snacking.

EVERYDAY STAPLES SHOPPING LIST

For suggestions on how much to buy, see "Organizing the Everyday Pantry and Spice Rack" in chapter 3 (page 55). Visit the "Resources" section for mail order links and recommended favorites (see page 320).

EVERYDAY SHOPPING LIST

VEGETABLES	GRAINS	Coconut oil	Coriander seed	Tongue scraper,
Beets	White basmati rice	Flax oil	Cumin seed	copper or
Carrots		Flaxseeds	Fennel seed	stainless steel
Collards	BEANS	Hemp seeds	Ginger powder	Tulsi tea
Kale	Mung beans,	Olive oil	Gingerroot	Vegetable broth
Parsley, fresh	green	Sunflower seeds	Pink salt	(when home-
Swiss chard	Mung beans,	Yogurt, fresh,	Sea salt	made isn't
	split yellow	whole milk	Turmeric	available, use
FRUITS				boxed broth,
Apples, in season	FATS	SPICES	EXTRAS	tamari, Bragg
Lemons	Almonds, raw	Cardamom	Ginger tea	Liquid Aminos,
Pears, in season	Butter, unsalted	powder	Honey, raw	bouillon cubes,
	(to make ghee)	Cinnamon	(except in	or Better than
	Chia seeds	powder	summer, see	Bouillon)
			page 129)	

Understanding the Everyday Recipes

The Everyday recipes on the pages that follow include boxes showing seasonal substitutions and additions. These variations will introduce the following qualities to balance each season.

KEY SEASONAL QUALITIES

SPRING	SUMMER	FALL	WINTER
Warming, light, dry	Cooling, dry, light	Grounding, moist, soft, slightly oily	Warming, grounding, moist, oily

WHY BUY ORGANIC?

For Your Body

In general, soft-skinned fruits and vegetables (like berries, grapes, apples, peaches, and tomatoes) have the greatest likelihood of carrying high levels of chemical residues, which can't be washed off. These chemicals can build up in your body over time, disturbing its natural intelligence and leading to accumulation of ama, the underlying cause of all disease.

For Everybody

The choices you make when you shop have far-reaching consequences. Supporting the industry of organic farming ensures that your food will be produced with kindness for the landscape, for your body, and for the farmers and their communities. If you are waffling, get on board with buying organic—just do it. All the money you save on eating out when you begin to prepare more of your own food is well spent on buying organic food!

On a Budget

The Environmental Working Group publishes annual lists of conventional (nonorganic) foods with the highest and lowest amounts of pesticide residue after washing. If your budget is tight at times, consult the EWG's "Dirty Dozen" and "Clean Fifteen" lists and choose organic when buying the foods on the first list (see "Resources," page 320).

WHY MUNG BEANS?

Ayurveda greatly favors the mung bean. The classic texts tell us the mung bean is light, beneficial for all body types, detoxifying, and easily digestible. You can use them in three varieties: sprouted, split with the skins removed, and whole. For more about sprouting mung beans, see Sprouted Mung Dal with Yogurt (page 261). I might eat mung dal two or three times a week in one of these forms, choosing between green, yellow, creamy, or crunchy dishes. Check the photo glossary (page 307) to see what mung beans look like whole and split.

everyday creamed grain cereal

serves 2

With just an immersion hand blender and some almond milk, you can turn plain grain into a special, nourishing breakfast. By changing the grain you use seasonally, you can change the qualities you start your day with, yet still enjoy a quick, hot breakfast. This recipe is a great way to use up extra cooked grain from another meal. For inspiration check out Berry Buck-Up Cereal (page 128) and Creamy Coconut Breakfast Barley with Peaches (page 173).

2 cups cooked grain of choice

1 cup almond milk or water

2–3 tbsp dried fruit (raisins, dates, dried cranberries) or seeds (sunflower, flax, hemp)

2 tsp Everyday Sweet Spice Mix (see page 118)

In a small saucepan, combine the cooked grain, milk or water, dried fruit, if using, and spice mix. Cover and warm the mixture on medium-low heat for 5 minutes. When it begins to steam, turn off the heat and use a hand blender to cream the cereal to the consistency you want—either smooth or still with some whole grains to look at and chew on. Do not overblend, as this will give the cereal a gummy texture.

Transfer to a breakfast bowl for serving. If adding seeds instead of fruit, sprinkle them on top as a garnish. Do not cook flax or hemp seeds, as the oils they contain are heat sensitive.

SEASONAL CREAMED GRAIN CEREALS

To vary your Everyday Creamed Grain Cereal by season, follow the method above, substituting the following seasonally appropriate ingredients:

MEASUREMENTS	SPRING	SUMMER	FALL	WINTER
2 cups cooked grain	Amaranth or rye	Quinoa or barley	Oats or bulgur wheat	Oats or bulgur wheat
1 cup liquid	Water	Water	Almond milk	Cow milk
3 tbsp mix-in	Raisins or chopped prunes, or flaxseeds	Sliced peaches or blueberries plus ½ tsp ground fennel seeds	Grated apple, dried apricots, or chopped almonds	Grated apple and/ or chopped dates
1 tsp fat	No	No	Ghee or coconut oil	Ghee
2 tsp spice mix	No	No	Sweet Spice Mix	Sweet Spice Mix

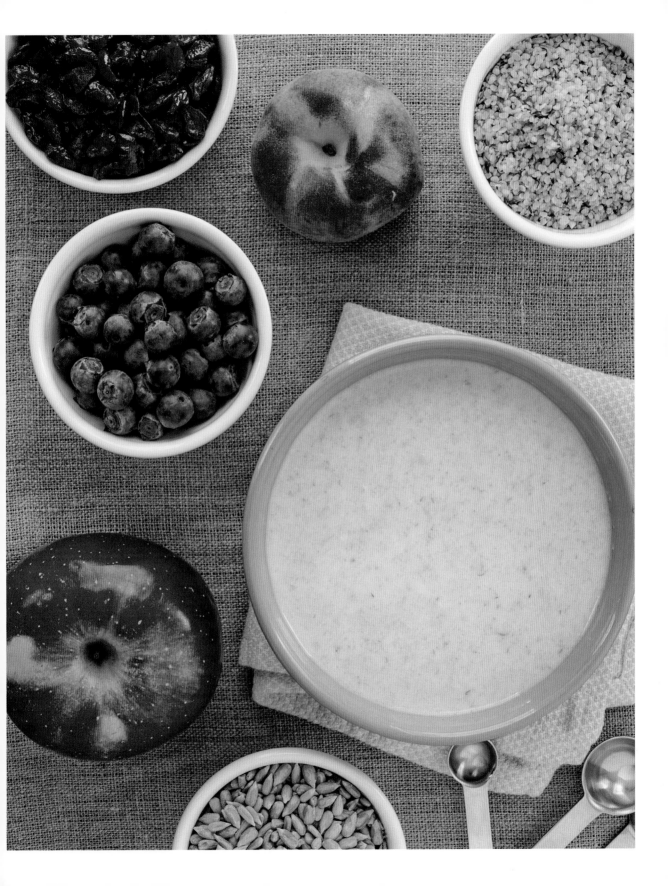

everyday chia pudding

serves 2

Chia seeds do not appear in traditional Ayurveda recipes, but their benefits are many. I eat them several times a week. Chia is a moist and grounding food, containing good fats, fiber, and a lubricating quality—a combination to remedy sluggish digestion. From an Ayurvedic perspective, the deeply hydrating action of chia seeds encourages life-supporting ojas (see page 31) and balances the degenerative nature of the dry quality by keeping the internal membranes moist—especially important in the dry times of year.

3 tbsp chia seeds
1 cup almond milk

MIX-INS:
Add one or more of
the following for flavor:
1–2 tsp maple syrup
1 tsp Everyday Sweet Spice Mix
   (see page 118)
½ tsp pure vanilla extract

Soak the chia seeds in almond milk for 5 minutes or more. Put the seeds, almond milk, and mix-ins in a blender carafe and blend on high speed for 2 minutes. The longer and faster you blend the pudding, the lighter and smoother it will be. You can use a hand blender, but the pudding will come out less smooth and fluffy.

Let the mixture stand for a few minutes to thicken before serving in bowls.

SHAKE IT UP: You can halve the amount of chia seeds to make this less of a pudding and more like a thick shake. You can also shake the mixture in a jar, not using a blender at all. This will yield a thick, tapioca-style pudding—and it's very convenient.

SEASONAL CHIA PUDDINGS

Follow the method above using the following ingredients and mix-ins to make seasonal chia pudding:

MEASUREMENTS	SPRING	SUMMER	FALL	WINTER
2 tbsp chia seeds	✓	✓	✓	✓
1 cup liquid	Pomegranate juice	Coconut water	Almond milk	Almond milk, warmed
Sweetener	1 tsp honey, 3 soaked prunes, or ¼ tsp stevia extract	1 tsp coconut sugar, 1 chopped date, or ¼ tsp stevia extract	2 tsp maple syrup, 2 chopped dates, or 2 tsp coconut sugar	½ tsp molasses or 2 chopped dates
Spice mix-in	1 tsp freshly grated ginger	no	1 tsp Everyday Sweet Spice Mix	1 tsp freshly grated ginger
Additional mix-ins (if desired)	1 cup fresh berries	1 cup blueberries, sprig of fresh mint	½ cup cooked squash, 1 tsp coconut oil, shredded coconut to taste	½ cup sweet potato puree, 1 tbsp nut butter, or 1 tbsp soaked cashews

See Pumpkin Chia Pudding (page 234) for my favorite seasonal pudding recipe.

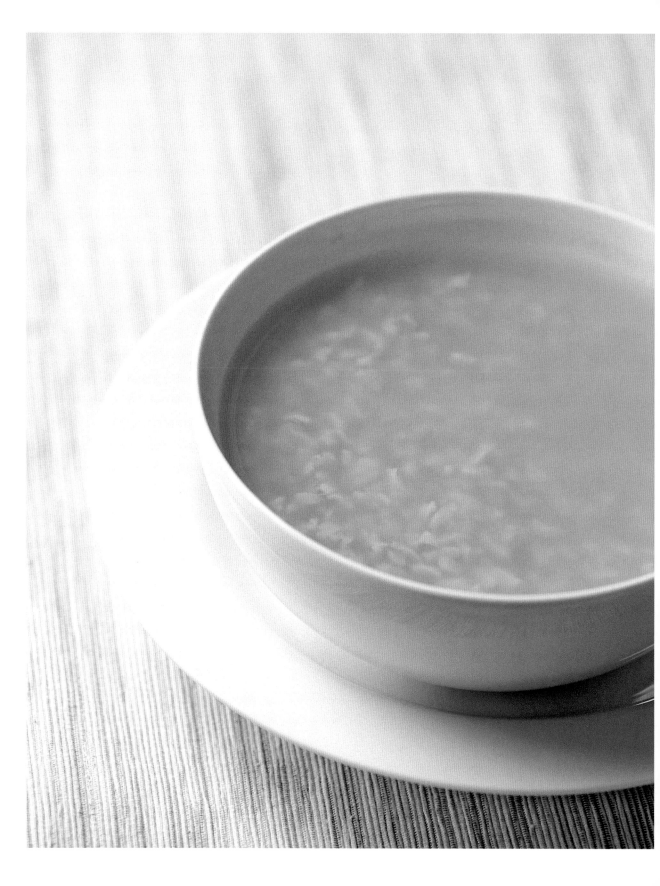

everyday kanjee

serves 4

Kanjee, also spelled *kanji*, means "gruel," and it can be prepared using different local grains, depending on the region of India. Kanjee is the absolute all-the-time healing food. Traditionally and to this day, in Ayurveda clinics and hospitals, practitioners nurse a patient's ailing digestion back to health by feeding her kanjee of increasing thickness as she begins to feel better. I find I crave kanjee the day after an indulgent meal, and a simple bowl gets me right back on track. If you eat this comfort food periodically, you are giving your digestion a break and are lessening the likelihood of experiencing signs and symptoms of imbalance.

For short-term fasting, strain the rice grains out and drink the kanjee water throughout the day. For everyday purposes, I suggest eating kanjee as a very simple breakfast or light dinner, choosing different grains for each season, if you like.

1 cup brown basmati rice, well rinsed

8 cups water

pinch each of salt, turmeric, and ginger powder

In a large saucepan, boil the water, salt, and spices on high heat. Add the rice to the pan. Allow the water to come to a boil again, then turn down the heat. Cover the rice and simmer for 1 hour, until the grains begin to split.

Ladle 2 cups of kanjee into each bowl for serving.

SEASONAL KANJEES

Follow the recipe for Everyday Kanjee, substituting the following grains for the rice and using these alternative spices:

MEASUREMENTS	SPRING	SUMMER	FALL	WINTER
1 cup grain, uncooked	Buckwheat, barley, rye, or millet	Quinoa or barley	Amaranth, quinoa, or oats	Wheat berries or oat groats
8 cups water	✓	✓	✓	✓
Spices	½ tsp freshly grated ginger and ½ tsp fenugreek seeds	1 tsp fennel seeds	2 tsp Everyday Sweet Spice Mix (optional)	Pinch each of cumin powder and cinnamon
Dried fruit	No	1 tbsp raisins	No	2 dates, chopped

everyday frittata

serves 4-6

This version of the classic baked-egg dish does not contain cheese, as in Ayurveda mixed eggs and dairy products are considered too heavy to digest well together. Goat cheese, however, has lighter and warmer qualities than cow's cheese, and I've included it as an addition for cool weather and for those who digest complicated foods well. Egg whites can be used in this recipe and are indicated for those with acid stomach or when heavy, dense qualities predominate in the body. For a smaller frittata, halve the recipe, cook it in a 6- to 8-inch skillet, and reduce the cooking time by as much as half.

1 tbsp ghee

2 cups vegetables, chopped into bite-size pieces (especially hearty greens, or choose from the seasonal fillings in the table below)

12 eggs

½ tsp salt

¼ tsp black pepper

½ tsp turmeric powder

Melt ghee in an 10- to 12-inch skillet on medium heat. (Cast-iron skillets are great for frittatas.) Stir in the vegetables and cook for 7-10 minutes, until tender. In a bowl, whisk the eggs, salt, pepper, and turmeric briskly with a fork for 1-2 minutes. Pour the egg mixture into the skillet with the vegetables. Cook over medium-low heat until eggs are almost set, about 8-10 minutes. To check, cut a small slit in the center of the frittata; when almost set, a small amount of uncooked egg will run into the cut. Cover and cook for 5-7 minutes more, or until eggs are completely set.

Right in the pan, cut into wedges for serving or turn whole onto a plate for presentation. This dish pairs well with steamed greens or with Cleansing Green Soup (see page 108).

EGGS AND AYURVEDA

Traditionally, eggs are cooked with a pinch each of turmeric and black pepper to help the body digest the heavy egg yolk. A warm, baked egg dish is preferable to a cold hard-boiled egg or an egg fried in lots of oil. In general, traditional Ayurveda considers eggs to increase heat and encourage excitability. Thus, they are not recommended for daily consumption but, rather, can be eaten one to four times a week, depending on the heat of your internal and external environments. (What's that mean? Read "Understanding Internal Climate," page 68.)

SEASONAL FRITTATAS

Customize the Everyday Frittata for each season with any combination of the seasonal vegetables listed below. Note that spinach and arugula do not need to be precooked. Simply stir chopped greens into the egg mixture before pouring into the skillet.

MEASUREMENTS	SPRING	SUMMER	FALL	WINTER
2 cups vegetables, chopped	Brussels sprouts, fiddleheads, asparagus, artichoke hearts, broccoli, arugula, spinach	Broccoli, summer squash, zucchini, cauliflower	Carrots, Brussels sprouts, kale, spinach	Carrots, kale, collards, chard
2 tsp ghee	✓	✓	✓	✓
8 eggs	✓	✓	✓	✓
½ tsp salt	✓	✓	✓	✓
¼ tsp black pepper	✓	✓	✓	✓
½ tsp turmeric	✓	✓	✓	✓
Extras			Top with 2 oz crumbled goat cheese after the eggs have begun to set	Add, with the vegetables: ¼ cup sliced olives and ¼ cup chopped tomato (for color)

everyday cream of anything soup

serves 2

Cream-based vegetable soups are moist, grounding, soft, and smooth. These qualities balance the erratic vibration of a busy schedule. A simple creamy soup—prepared with or without traditional dairy products—helps support you through a big day.

If you follow the seasonal shopping lists in this book, you will have a few choices of "cream" bases on hand. Learn the basic technique described below, and in a short time, you will find a couple of favorite staples that will keep you enjoying your own cooking.

LUNCH

4 cups water or vegetable broth

4 cups of chopped kale, collard greens, Swiss chard, and/or carrots

2 tsp Everyday Savory Spice Mix (see page 117) or Everyday Digestive Salts (see page 118)

½ tsp turmeric powder

1-inch piece fresh gingerroot, peeled

2 tsp ghee

1 cup almond milk

In a medium saucepan over high heat, bring the water or broth to a boil. Add the vegetables, spice mix or salts, turmeric, and gingerroot to the saucepan, reduce heat, and simmer, covered, for about 10 minutes. The longer you let it cook, the creamier your soup will be; less time means your soup will have a thicker texture and your vegetables will be more al dente. Fresh greens, like baby spinach, take only a few minutes to wilt, whereas for harder vegetables, like celery and carrots, I'd recommend the full 10-minute cooking time or even longer. If you like your soup very creamy, simmer your greens and the hard vegetables, like carrots, an extra 5 minutes.

Transfer the vegetables in their cooking liquid to a blender carafe. Add the ghee and the almond milk—the latter will cool the mixture down to keep your blender from getting too hot. Blend on medium to start, then high until smooth. Alternatively, use an immersion hand blender and process the soup right in the saucepan, along with the ghee and almond milk, until smooth.

The soup should be warm enough to serve right away. Ladle into 2 large bowls and dig in. This soup pairs well with Everyday Dosa on the side.

SEASONAL CREAMED VEGETABLE SOUPS

Follow the method above, substituting with these seasonal ingredients:

MEASUREMENTS	SPRING	SUMMER	FALL	WINTER
4 cups water or vegetable broth	✓	✓	✓	✓
4 cups veggies	Asparagus, celery, mustard greens, green beans, spinach	Summer squash, fennel bulbs, green beans	Green beans, kale, chard, squash, carrots, beets	Dark leafy greens, sweet potatoes, carrots, beets, parsnips
2 tsp Spice Mix or Salts	Spring	Summer	Fall	Winter
½ tsp turmeric powder	✓	✓	✓	✓
1-inch fresh gingerroot, peeled	✓	✓	✓	✓
2 tsp fat	Ghee, sunflower oil, or grapeseed oil	Ghee, coconut oil, sunflower oil	Ghee, coconut oil, or olive oil	Ghee, sesame oil, or olive oil
1 cup milk	1 cup white beans or cooked cauliflower to replace milk	White beans, 8 oz silken tofu, coconut milk, or cooked cauliflower	Cow, goat, coconut, or 8 oz silken tofu	Cow, goat, ½ cup soaked cashews blended with ½ cup water, or 8 oz silken tofu

For some tasty alternatives, check out Surprising Cream of Broccoli Soup (page 227) and Asparagus and White Bean Soup (page 136).

everyday steamed salad bowl

serves 2

I'd like to see everyone get in the habit of eating more cooked food. Food that is warm, soft, and moist is easier on the gut than raw food and very grounding for the system. The busier your day is, the less appropriate a raw or cold meal will be for your body—whatever the weather. In this foundational recipe, I suggest eating colorful piles of steamed vegetables over bowls of grains or proteins, augmented with dressings and sauces, all year-round. Steaming vegetables reduces their volume, making it easy for you to get a medicinal share of veggies.

Accent your steamed vegetables with seasonal bean pâtés, cooked grains, chutneys, a sprinkle of Mineral Gomasio (page 265), or any of the sauces and spreadables from the seasonal chapters—this will bring variety to your rotating cast of seasonal vegetables (for a quick list, see appendix 2, "Seasonal Shopping Lists," on page 304). Toasted sunflower seeds work well any time of year. In addition, in the "Seasonal Steamed Salad Bowls" on page 96, I have included specific seasonal proteins to bulk up your steamed salad and make it a complete meal.

4 leaves lacinato kale

6 leaves rainbow Swiss chard

2 carrots

½ cup chopped red cabbage

½ cup sprouted mung beans (see page 262)

2 cups cooked basmati rice, white or brown

All-Seasons Salad Dressing

handful toasted sunflower seeds

Remove the stems from the kale and chard and chop the leaves into 2-inch pieces. Place the greens in a large frying pan with 1 tbsp of water. Tightly cover the greens and steam sauté for 10 minutes.

Using a vegetable peeler or julienne peeler, slice the carrots into ribbons. Add to the steam sauté, along with the chopped cabbage and sprouted mung beans. Steam 5 minutes more. Remove from the heat and leave the lid slightly ajar.

Make beds of rice in 2 wide bowls or plates by spreading 1 cup of rice over the bottom of each bowl. Divide the steamed vegetables on top of the rice. Pour half of the All-Seasons Salad Dressing over each serving and sprinkle with toasted sunflower seeds.

ALL-SEASONS SALAD DRESSING

½ cup fresh lemon juice

¼ cup cold-pressed olive oil

1 tsp Everyday Digestive Salts (see page 118) or 1 tsp salt plus 1 tsp Everyday Savory Spice Mix (see page 117)

dash of pepper

Shake all the ingredients together in a pint-size jar. Keeps in the refrigerator for up to 5 days.

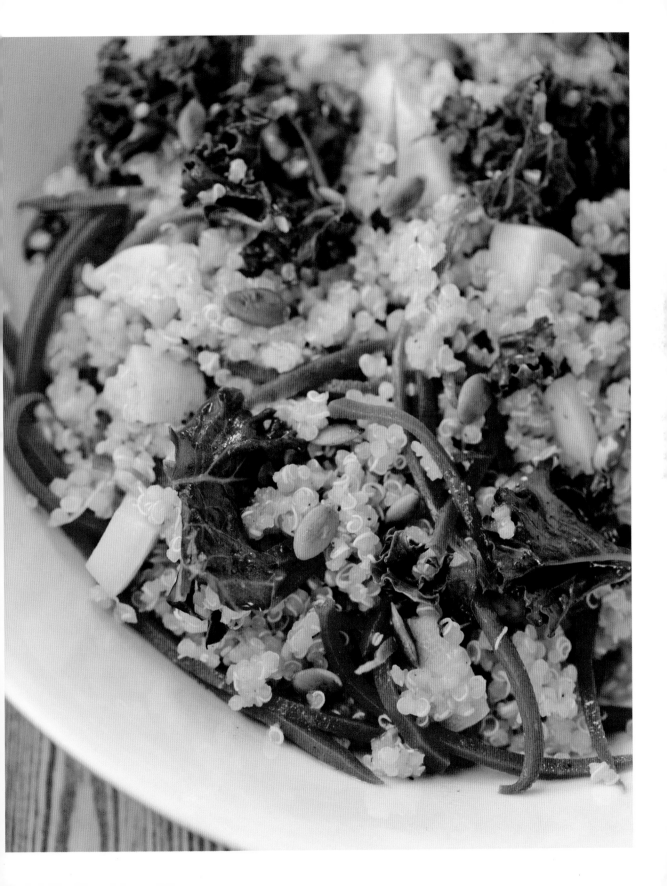

SEASONAL STEAMED SALAD BOWLS

Follow the above method, replacing the vegetables, proteins, and dressings as shown in the seasonal table below. For the winter variation, which calls for nuts, please note that nuts can be chopped for sprinkling on top or served whole and crunchy.

MEASUREMENTS	SPRING	SUMMER	FALL	WINTER
4 cups veggies	Radicchio, arugula, dandelion greens, endive, Brussels sprouts, broccoli, asparagus	Cauliflower, broccoli, celery, okra, green beans, zucchini, summer squash	Squash, collards, spinach, peas, green beans, sweet potatoes, beets, carrot	Sweet potatoes, collards, spinach, squash, tomatoes, beets, carrots
2 cups grain	Barley	Quinoa	Quinoa	Bulgur wheat
Dressing	Mustard Balsamic Vinaigrette (see page 163)	Cilantro Mint Chutney (see page 202)	Whipped Tahini Sauce (see page 217)	Miso Sesame Dressing (see page 287)
Toppings	Cooked egg white, hemp seeds, dried cherries, or nutritional yeast flakes	Hemp seeds or nutritional yeast flakes	Poached egg, Mineral Gomasio (see page 265), or Ume Pumpkin Seeds (see page 228)	Poached egg or a handful of meaty nuts such as cashews, hazelnuts, brazil nuts, macadamia nuts, or Roasted Maple Almonds (see page 269)

SEASONAL FOOD PYRAMID

What is the easiest and best way to know which produce is in season (besides shopping at a farmers' market, where all the food is locally grown and freshly harvested)? When you walk into a grocery store, you'll often see a few pyramids overflowing with an abundance of fruits or vegetables and *on sale*. If an item is on sale and on prominent display, you know it is plentiful right now. Shop the sale pyramids for seasonal success!

everyday dosa

makes about 12

Every culture has its crepe, pancake, tortilla, or flatbread. India gives us the gift of dosa, which bears most resemblance to France's crepe. Dosa is traditionally served with a spicy soup and chutney. This flatbread is most often made with polished or parboiled white rice and split urad dal, which is a hulled pigeon pea. This recipe calls for split mung dal and white basmati rice; both are light and dry in quality yet grounding and nourishing when soaked, cooked, and served warm. Adventurous cooks may replace the mung dal with urad dal, which is highly nutritive and heavier, making it a great variation for cooler weather. Unlike the other Everyday recipes, which feature seasonal variations, this simple dosa recipe can be served as a year-round staple.

A steaming hot dosa pairs well with both savory and sweet dishes. Dosa can be eaten with ghee (especially if you need to balance the dry quality) and maple syrup in winter, with Notella Hazelnut Spread (see page 148) to satisfy a spring sweet tooth, or with sweetened coconut milk in summer.

NOTE: This recipe requires overnight soaking, so plan ahead.

1 cup white basmati rice

1 cup split yellow mung beans

1¼ cup fresh water

½ tsp salt

½ tsp coriander powder (optional)

coconut oil for frying

Using a large mixing bowl and fine mesh sieve, wash and strain the rice and the mung beans twice or until the water runs clear. Transfer the rice and mung beans to a 4-quart saucepan or mixing bowl. Cover the mixture with fresh water and soak for at least 6 hours or overnight. After the soaking period, strain and rinse the rice and mung beans.

Next, grind the rice and mung beans. If using a large food processor, put all the rice and beans in the processor bowl, add the water, salt, and coriander, and grind on high for 5 minutes. If using a blender, put half of the water and about half of the rice and beans in the blender carafe and blend on high for 1 minute. Then gradually add more of the rice and beans until the mixture becomes like pancake batter, blending on high for at least 3 minutes. If your blender gets hot, stop. You may have to process the recipe in two batches.

Return the batter to a bowl or saucepan, cover with a towel, and leave it somewhere warm to ferment for 8–12 hours or overnight. If you live in a cool climate, putting it on top of the fridge or in the oven (don't turn it on) will work.

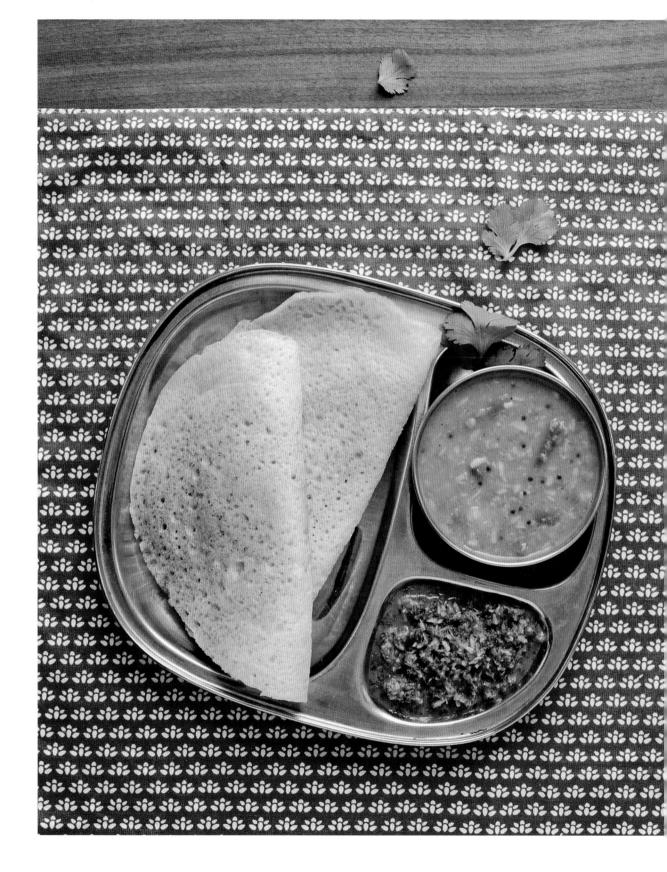

Fermentation will make the batter rise in the bowl. The more the dough ferments, the lighter and fluffier the dosa.

Warm a ceramic nonstick frying pan over medium heat and use ½ tsp coconut oil per dosa (or a spray coconut oil) in the pan. Flick a few drops of water on the pan's surface; when the water sizzles the pan is ready. Cook the dosa as you would a pancake. Pour ⅓ cup of the dosa batter into the pan. Tilt and rotate the pan to spread the batter out evenly. If your batter is very thick, use the back of a large spoon to spread it in circles until the dosa is thin.

When the dosa bubbles and the edges start to come away from the pan, check to see that the bottom is nice and brown. It's done. If you like your dosa crisp, flip it and cook a few minutes more. Each dosa takes about 5 minutes.

For a traditional pairing, serve with a small bowl of South Indian Sambar (page 132) for dipping and perhaps a side of Cilantro Mint Chutney (page 202). You will find Everyday Dosa goes well with many soups and sauces in this book.

FAMILY-STYLE DOSA

Homemade dosa is a real treat to share. You can prepare a few and keep them stacked in a warm oven until you have enough to serve. In Indian households, whoever is cooking will stay in the kitchen preparing dosa and bring them out one at time to the family or guests. The cook keeps them coming, and in between the folks at the table are resting and socializing. The meal goes on until everyone has had enough of dosa. I've seen the man of the house eat six!

everyday kichari

serves 4–6

Kichari is the balancing staple food of Ayurveda. Served regularly at Ayurveda clinics and centers, this is a neutral, light, and soft food that both cleanses and nourishes the body, without supporting imbalance of any kind. In fact, kichari is thought to remove toxins from the system. This complete, one-pot meal is a mixture of hulled mung beans and rice, known to be gentle on the digestive organs, cooked with a rotating cast of vegetables and spices. Once you get the hang of the formula, you can experiment with seasonal varieties of beans and grains. Most would do well to eat this dish three to four times a week; I do, and it feels great.

6   cups water

1   cup basmati rice

½   cup yellow split mung dal (ideally, soaked for 1 hour or more)

1 tbsp Everyday Savory Spice Mix (see page 117)

pinch of asafetida (hing) powder (optional)

2   cups vegetables (choose from the Everyday Shopping List in appendix 2, page 304), coarsely chopped into ½-inch cubes, leafy greens also coarsely chopped into strips

½–1 tsp salt

fresh cilantro for garnish

FOR THE TEMPERING

1–2 tbsp ghee

½ tsp cumin seed

½ tsp coriander seed

½ tsp fennel seed (optional)

In a large saucepan boil 5 cups water on high heat. Set the other 1 cup aside to add during cooking as needed.

Rinse the rice and dal twice or until water runs clear. Add them to the boiling water, along with the spice mix and optional hing, and keep on high heat until the liquid boils again. Then immediately turn the heat down to low. If using hard vegetables like potatoes, carrots, and squash, add the ½-inch cubes now. Partially cover the pan with the lid ajar and simmer for 20 minutes without stirring. Check after 20 minutes to see if it needs more water. If the dal is not submerged, it does. Pour the additional cup of water on top and do not stir. If using quick-cooking vegetables like greens, green beans, and the like, add those on top to steam now. Simmer partially covered 10 minutes more.

To make the tempering, warm the ghee in a small skillet on medium heat. Add the cumin, coriander, and optional fennel seeds and cook until the seeds pop, about 2–3 minutes. Remove from heat and pour into the kichari. Add salt, stir well, and let stand, covered, for a few minutes.

Kichari should have a soupy, soft consistency; serve it in bowls, as you would a stew. Garnish with fresh cilantro.

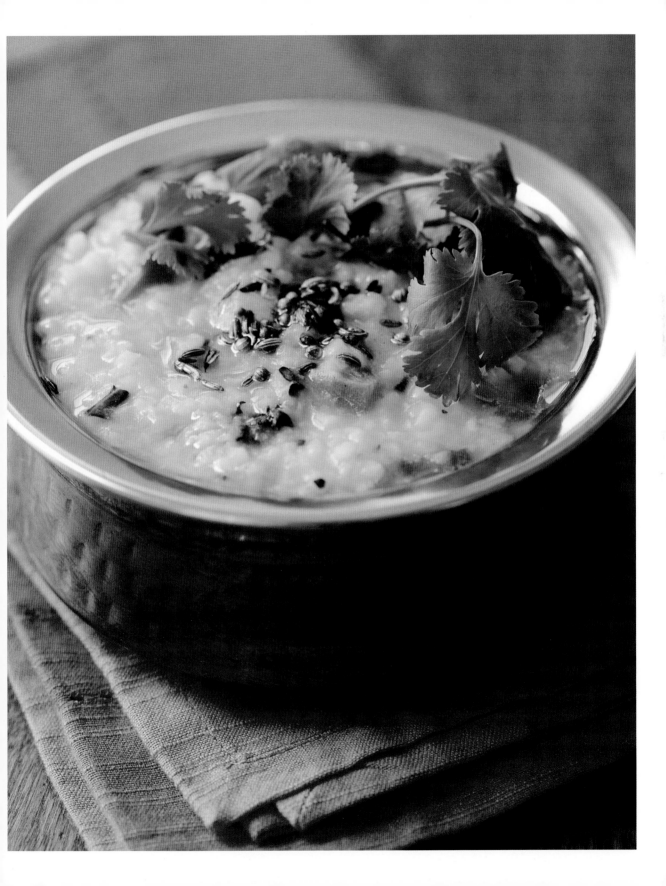

SEASONAL KICHARIS

Follow the Everyday Kichari recipe on page 100, substituting these seasonal variations:

MEASUREMENTS	SPRING	SUMMER	FALL	WINTER
6 cups water	✓	✓	✓	✓
1 cup basmati rice	✓	✓	✓	✓
½ cup yellow split mung dal	✓	✓	✓	✓
1 tbsp Spice Mix	Spring	Summer	Fall	Winter
Pinch of hing	✓	✓	✓	✓
2 cups veggies (choose one)	Arugula, dandelion greens, endive, cabbage, Brussels sprouts, broccoli, asparagus, sprouted mung beans	Cauliflower, broccoli, celery, okra, green beans, zucchini and summer squash, sprouted mung beans	Pumpkin, squash, kale, collards, chard, spinach, peas, green beans, sweet potatoes, carrots, sea vegetables	Sweet potatoes, kale, collards, chard, spinach, squash, carrots, sea vegetables
Tempering	✓	Yes; you may substitute coconut oil for the ghee	✓	✓
½ –1 tsp salt	✓	✓	✓	✓
Garnish	Squeeze of lemon	Fresh lime wedges or fresh herbs such as parsley, basil, or thyme leaves	Add shredded coconut to tempering and toast for 1 minute	Drizzle additional 1 tsp melted ghee over top

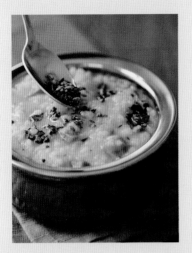

Keep it simple: Season with just the spice mix and add ghee to each bowl for serving.

Make it special: The longer you cook it, the more wonderful it tastes, and the easier it is to digest. You could simmer the kichari for about 1 hour. In this case, simmer the rice and mung beans, covered, for as much as 40 minutes. Then add the harder vegetables for the last 20 minutes, and steam quick-cooking vegetables on top for only the last 10 or so minutes. Check in about halfway through, because you may need a cup or two more of hot water to keep your kichari soft. You can also make kichari ahead in a slow cooker or rice cooker, and you will have food when you come home from work.

Veggie tip: The more finely you chop your vegetables, the faster they will cook. Half-inch cubes of a hard winter vegetable cook in 20–25 minutes. Baby spinach or arugula, which is naturally fine, can be stirred in with the tempering toward the end.

WHAT ARE FOOD SENSITIVITIES?

What we in the West know as food intolerance or sensitivities, Ayurveda views as a result of poor digestion and elimination. Symptoms such as acid indigestion, gas and bloating, loose stools, or constipation may result when a body isn't tolerating a food well. Generally, weak agni and/or incomplete elimination allow toxicity to build up in the body. This leads to a sensitivity, or in some cases intolerance, especially to sticky, hard-to-digest foods, like wheat and dairy products. Gunked-up organs are unable to break down certain foods, so the body rejects them or they remain undigested, leading to the creation of ama, more toxicity in the body. A number of factors—which depend very much on the individual—have an impact on food sensitivities. Impaired digestive fire can result from:

- not digesting a substance well or ingesting a substance too often
- taking in too great a quantity at one time
- eating at the wrong time of day
- processing: modern processing and genetic engineering may be creating substances that are unfamiliar to the body and indigestible, so the body rejects them.

The Ayurvedic approach to food sensitivities begins with strengthening the digestive fire. Kichari is just the food to help a reactive system rest and recover. To learn how to care for your digestive fire, see chapter 2, "The Principles of Ayurvedic Eating."

everyday basmati rice

Basmati rice is a staple side dish and the center of any Ayurvedic meal because of its sweet taste and cooling effect. I find quick-cooking basmati nicely rounds out a cleansing green soup or dal, and I eat it once or twice a week. Basmati rice is prized for its fragrance and light texture. Note how fine and long the uncooked grains are and how, in the final product, they remain delicate and light. White basmati is considered easy to assimilate and nourishing to all body types. Rinsing rice well removes extra starch, while soaking before cooking softens the grain a bit, ensuring a light and digestible Everyday Basmati Rice.

LUNCH

1 cup white basmati rice

2 cups water

¼ tsp ghee

¼ tsp salt

Using a fine mesh sieve, rinse the rice under cool, running water. Submerge the sieve, rice and all, in a bowl of cool water, allowing rice to soak for 30 minutes. Drain the rice and rinse one last time under cool running water until the water runs clear.

Add the rice to a medium-size saucepan with the water, the ghee (which keeps the pot from boiling over and balances the dry quality of the grain), and the salt. Bring to a boil over medium high heat. Cover, reduce heat to low, and simmer for 17 minutes. Do not disturb the rice while it cooks—no peeking under the lid or stirring! After 17 minutes, remove it from heat and let it stand for 5 minutes with the lid on.

Remove the lid, fluff with a fork, and serve.

WHITE RICE OR BROWN?

The fibrous bran from the hull is left on brown rices and removed in white rices. In India, when the tall shafts of rice are harvested, farmers have traditionally put them in the road so that passing trucks drive over the grain and break off the husks. The nutritious bran remains stuck to the grain, which we know as brown rice. When the bran is peeled off, the rice is "polished" or white.

Although Western health movements suggest that only brown rice is beneficial, Ayurveda considers white basmati (not parboiled or short grain) rice easier to digest than brown, especially when one's digestive fire is not strong enough to digest the hull well or when one has a sensitive or inflamed digestive tract, for which fiber can be too rough.

Traditionally, Ayurveda makes mention of many varieties of local grains. Black millet, called *ragi*, and red rice are two grains I have enjoyed in southern India. While the average palate is used to eating white rice in India, I am seeing a movement toward a return to whole grains for health, supported by Ayurvedic wisdom.

SEASONAL RECIPES AND ROUTINES

everyday bean pâté

serves 4

Beans are generally dry, astringent, and light. This makes them a good choice for encouraging weight loss and alleviating water retention—but if your body is on the dry side, add a bit more oil and salt to your pâtés. In Ayurveda canned beans are considered stale, but home-cooked, pureed beans are smooth, soft, and easy to digest, as well as versatile. Each seasonal bean pâté contains a bean, an oil, a salt, a spice, and something with zing. Beans add protein to any wrap (like the Collard Wraps with Red Lentil Pâté, see page 267), an Everyday Steamed Salad Bowl, or a simple grain.

1 cup cooked red lentils

½–1 cup water

1 tsp Everyday Savory Spice Mix (see page 117)

½ tsp red miso

1 tsp olive oil

1 tsp fresh lemon juice

Place the cooked lentils in a large mixing bowl and add ½ cup water, spice mix, miso, olive oil, and lemon juice. Depending how smooth you would like your pâté, either mash the ingredients together with a fork or mix with an electric hand blender until the texture is smooth. Add the remaining ½ cup water if needed to achieve desired consistency.

Serve this pâté beside an Everyday Steamed Salad Bowl; in a wrap made with collards, nori, or Everyday Dosa; or as a dip for parboiled vegetable spears or crackers.

Seasonal Bean Pâtés continue on page 107.

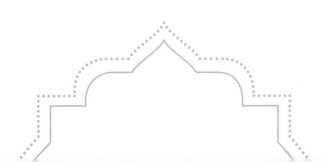

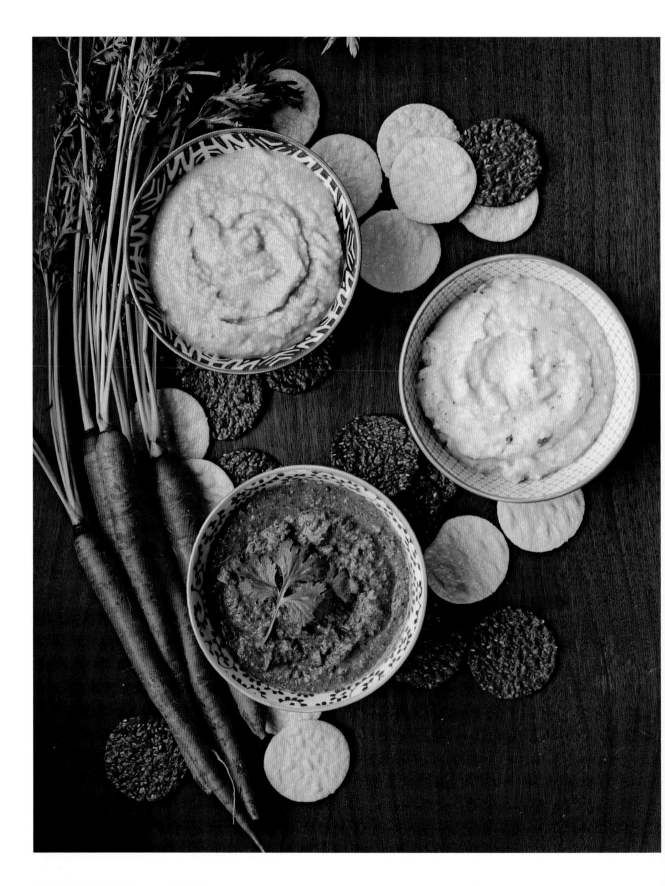

Create seasonal bean pâtés by following the Everyday method on page 105, substituting the ingredients in the table below.

MEASUREMENTS	SPRING	SUMMER	FALL	WINTER
1 cup cooked legumes	Red lentils	Split mung dal	Adzuki beans	Red lentils
½–1 cup water	✓	✓	✓	✓
1 tsp Spice Mix	Spring	Summer	Fall	Winter
½ tsp red miso	✓	✓	✓	✓
1 tsp fat	Grapeseed oil	Olive oil	Olive oil	Sesame oil
1 tsp lemon or vinegar	Apple cider vinegar	Fresh lemon juice	Fresh lemon juice	Rice vinegar
Additional spices/herbs	Dash of cayenne or chili powder	2 tbsp finely chopped fresh herbs (cilantro, basil, or parsley)	¼ tsp ginger powder	none
Serving suggestion	Wrap in collard greens or serve as a dip with parboiled vegetable spears.	Serve with rice crackers and raw vegetable spears.	Serve on sliced, roasted squash, or wrapped in Toasted Nori.	Serve with baked sweet potato wedges, rice, or sprouted grain toast.

For another spin on the bean pâté, see Spicy Black Bean Hummus (page 160) and Collard Wraps with Red Lentil Pâté (see page 267).

everyday cleansing green soup

serves 2–4

Everyday Cleansing Green Soup is a warm alternative to cold green juice. Green vegetables always contain astringent and bitter tastes. These two tastes, along with pungency, represent the reducing qualities in Ayurveda. This soup is indicated any time you need a break from heavy foods, want to lose some weight, or desire a lift for your digestion or mood. Eating Everyday Cleansing Green Soup is a great habit, and I have seen a number of clients fall in love with this soup.

SUPPER

3 cups vegetable broth

1 tsp turmeric powder

1-inch piece fresh gingerroot

1 cup packed chopped kale (about 2 small leaves)

4 cups packed chopped Swiss chard (about 4 large leaves)

1 cup packed parsley leaves, no stems (about 2 big handfuls)

2 tsp ghee or coconut oil

salt and pepper to taste

In a 2-quart saucepan, combine the vegetable broth and turmeric powder and bring to a boil on high heat. (If you plan to use a carafe blender, reserve 1 cup of the broth at room temperature to add later.) Peel and coarsely chop the gingerroot and add to the pot. Add the chopped kale and chard. Cover and simmer on medium heat for 10 minutes. Stir in the parsley and oil.

Remove from heat. If using an immersion hand blender, process in saucepan until completely smooth. If using a carafe blender, transfer liquid and vegetables to carafe and add the reserved cup of broth to cool the mixture down. Put a towel over the blender top and hold it down with your hand. Begin blending on low, gradually increasing the speed, until the soup is smooth. You may need to blend in two batches.

Enjoy this soup topped with toasted sunflower seeds; alongside Everyday Dosa or sprouted grain toast with ghee; or, in warm weather, with hummus and rye or rice crackers.

SEASONAL CLEANSING GREEN SOUPS

Follow the Everyday method above, using the seasonal ingredients listed in this table.

MEASUREMENTS	SPRING	SUMMER	FALL	WINTER
3 cups vegetable broth	✓	✓	✓	✓
1 tsp turmeric powder	✓	✓	✓	✓
1-inch piece of fresh gingerroot	✓	✓	✓	✓
1 cup packed chopped kale	✓	✓	✓	✓
4 cups packed chopped vegetables (any combination)	Broccoli, arugula, cabbage, Brussels sprouts, celery	Summer squash, zucchini, green beans, celery, broccoli	Spinach, peas, green beans	Spinach, Brussels sprouts, mung bean sprouts, cabbage
1 cup packed parsley leaves	✓	✓	✓	✓
2 tsp fat	Ghee or grapeseed oil	Coconut oil	Ghee or coconut oil	Ghee or coconut oil + ½–1 peeled avocado (optional)
Salt and pepper to taste	✓	✓	✓	✓

easy morning beverage

serves 1

As its name implies, this warm drink is recommended first thing in the morning. Lemon stimulates a cleansing flush by encouraging bile production, which will get things moving! The sharp quality of lemon breaks up mucus and any nighttime buildup in the stomach, but to balance this sharp quality, add a hint of sweet. In cold weather, make a winter warmer by boiling one teaspoon of grated gingerroot in the water before adding lemon.

1¼ cups water
juice of ¼ lemon
1 tsp dehydrated sugarcane
   (optional)

In a small pot or kettle, bring the water to a boil. Remove from heat and pour boiling water into a large mug.

To serve, stir in fresh-squeezed lemon juice and sweetener, if using.

COFFEE TALK

While we are on the topic of morning beverages . . . what does Ayurveda say about coffee?

Caffeine in any form is astringent, and astringent equals drying. You will notice you have a dry mouth after drinking coffee, black tea, and even green tea.

Coffee is heating, sharp, light, slightly oily, *and* drying. This heavy-hitting combo creates a hot and dry internal environment. The one time in my life I have deeply craved coffee was on the island of Kaua'i (which, incidentally, has great coffee). After a few days of absolutely still air and rain, the drying, light qualities of coffee felt like God's gift, as they balanced the weather pattern's insistently heavy, moist qualities. Coffee is strong medicine, though, and there are more sustainable ways to find a balance in your body.

I have seen clients have very good luck by reducing coffee intake slowly, one cup or half a cup at a time. In some cases a small cup each day is tolerable and worth the joie de vivre it brings. In other cases, I have seen clients abstain from coffee altogether by replacing the dark, bitter, roasted-bean beverage with roasted dandelion root, a plant native to Europe and the Americas and known to benefit the liver. I often hear people say drinking coffee is simply a habit, a ritual, as if they do not even care about the substance itself. Try substituting some roasted dandelion root coffee for your ritual. It contains the same qualities as regular coffee, without being sharp or dry.

Remember, it is when coffee begins sneaking in more than once a day or the one cup is gaining in ounces that you need to rein it in.

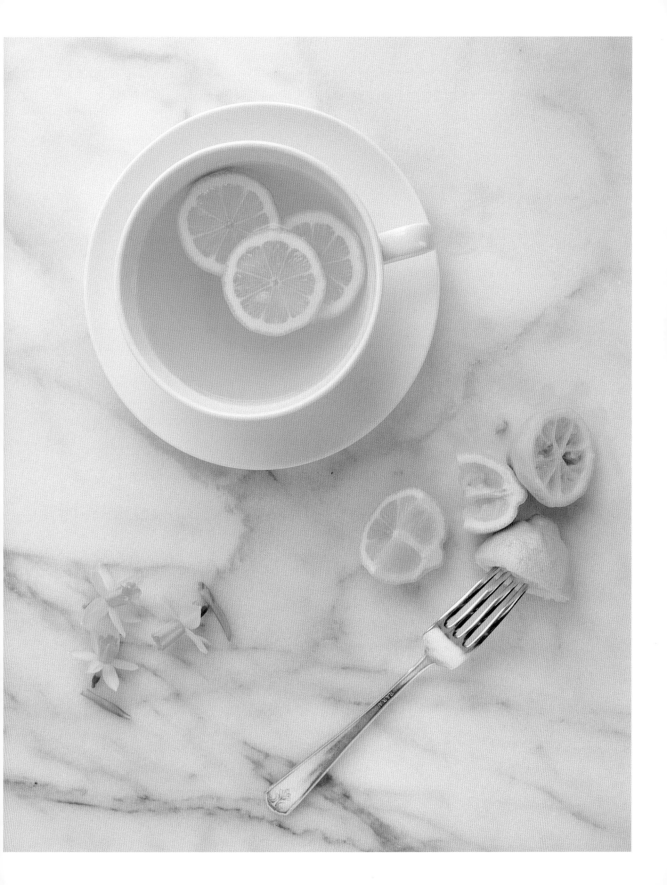

everyday digestive lassi

serves 2

The Ayurvedic lassi is quite different from the kind you find in Indian restaurants. A restaurant lassi is very thick and rich, made with undiluted yogurt, often blended with ice and banana or mango. This is not a digestive beverage; it's a gut-bomb! The medicinal way of drinking cultured milk is to dilute it with water and to skim off some of the fat. The weaker one's digestion is, the more fat one should remove. Churning the cultured milk with water introduces light, mobile qualities to whole fat milk, which is otherwise heavy, dense, and oily. For this recipe you can use yogurt or kefir, not the buttermilk sold in stores. Traditional lassi is a postdigestive probiotic, which settles the stomach and increases digestion and absorption of nutrients. Lassi is most strongly recommended after the midday meal.

1 cup water, room
    temperature
¼ cup organic whole milk
    yogurt
dash of turmeric powder
dash of ginger powder

Put the water in a 16-ounce glass jar and add the yogurt and spices. Churn the mixture on high speed for 1 minute with an immersion hand blender, until it foams. Some of the milk solids will gather on top and stick to the sides of the jar; they look like little bubbles. When the liquid settles, skim off the solids with a spoon and discard.

To serve, pour into two 8-ounce glasses.

FRESH, WHOLE MILK YOGURT

Ayurveda recommends eating fresh yogurt or drinking fresh kefir, as the longer a cultured dairy product has been sitting, the more sour its sweet taste becomes. If you are not making it at home, try to buy a locally made yogurt or kefir. Also, nonfat yogurt is more sour than yogurt made with whole milk, as its sweet taste is removed along with its fat. Choosing whole milk yogurt and separating the fats yourself by churning, as described in the recipe, will yield a more beneficial lassi than using nonfat yogurt.

SEASONAL DIGESTIVE LASSIS

Create seasonal variations by following the method above, using the ingredients in this table.

MEASUREMENTS	SPRING	SUMMER	FALL	WINTER
1 cup water, room temperature	✓	✓	✓	✓
¼ cup organic whole milk yogurt	✓	✓	✓	✓
Spices	Dash of turmeric and ginger powder + ¼ tsp ground coriander	Dash of cardamom powder and 4–6 mint leaves	¼ tsp cinnamon	Dash of turmeric and ginger powder
Sweetener	½ tsp raw honey	No	½ tsp maple syrup or coconut sugar	1 Medjool date, pitted and chopped

everyday almond milk

makes 1 quart

The Ayurvedic diet often includes almonds for their slightly cooling and nutritive action, which reaches all the tissue layers. Almonds are also thought to improve the skin and increase its luster and beauty. Apart from soaking time, fresh almond milk takes only a few minutes to make, and it offers far more vitality than the kind you buy in a box. Everyday Almond Milk is the base for many of the soups and baking recipes in this book; you might make up a quart every few days and save the leftover almond meal for baking. This recipe keeps well for 3–5 days in the refrigerator, but I am in the habit of making a half batch every other day. It tastes so delicious fresh!

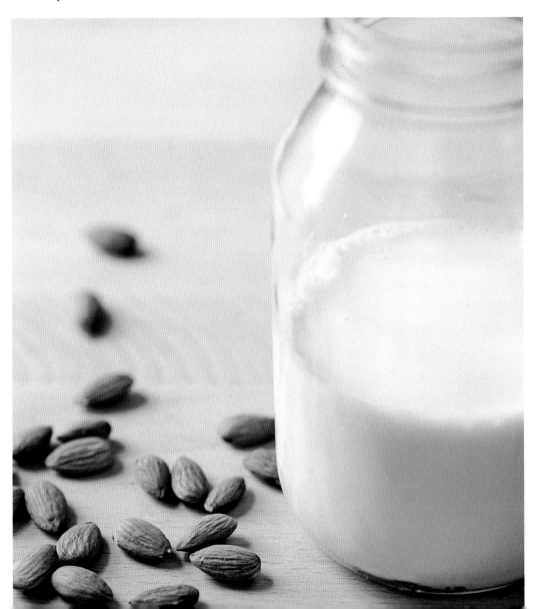

⅔ cup raw almonds

4 cups water, plus about 2 cups for soaking

dash of salt (optional)

Soak the almonds for 6 or more hours (overnight works) in enough water to cover, about 2 cups. Drain and discard the water and rinse the almonds. Using a hand blender or a carafe blender, process them with 1 cup of water until smooth. Add the remaining 3 cups of water. Blend again until smooth and foamy.

To serve or use for recipes, strain the milk through a fine sieve or cheesecloth (strain twice if you like it very smooth). Save the resulting pulp for baking or for thickening blended soups.

SEASONAL NUT MILK VARIATIONS

Milk made from soaked almonds is beneficial in all seasons, but you might also enjoy the following seasonal milk recipes. Follow the instructions for Everyday Almond Milk above, but note that with different ingredients the soaking times may change, as well as whether you use the soaking water in your milk or drain and rinse the nuts or seeds first.

MEASUREMENTS	SPRING	SUMMER	FALL	WINTER
⅔ cup nut or seed	Hemp seeds	Raw sunflower seeds	Steel cut oats	Raw cashews
Amount of water	2 cups, plus 1 cup for soaking	4 cups water, plus 2 cups for soaking	4 cups water, plus 2 cups for soaking	2 cups water, plus 2 cups for soaking
Dash of salt (optional)	no	✓	✓	✓
Soaking method	You need to soak hemp seeds for only 15 minutes. You may reuse the soaking water in the recipe.	Soak sunflower seeds overnight. Drain and rinse before using. Discard soak water.	Soak steel cut oats overnight. Drain and rinse well before using. Discard soak water.	Soak cashews 4–8 hours. You may reuse the soaking water in the recipe.

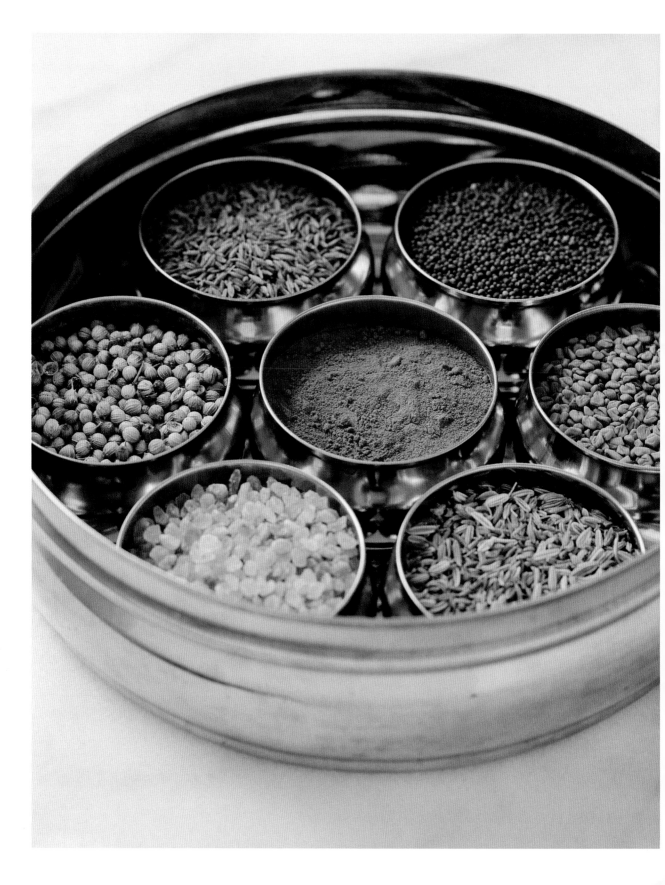

everyday ayurvedic spice mixes and salts

Two simple spice mixes, one sweet and one savory, are featured in many of the Everyday recipes and can come in quite handy in your other cookery or as condiments. Steamed vegetables topped with ghee and Everyday Savory Spice Mix need no special sauce. Cooked fruits or cereals with a dash of Everyday Sweet Spice Mix are ready to enjoy. The familiar taste of Everyday Digestive Salts can spruce up almost anything with minimal effort. Keep these mixes in your kitchen to enjoy their neutral, beneficial qualities for year-round eating and healing.

EVERYDAY SAVORY SPICE MIX

makes ¼ cup

The combination of turmeric, cumin, coriander, and fennel is a traditionally balanced digestive formula for kindling agni, stimulating liver function, and moderating the fire element. You will notice this mixture is the basis for all of the seasonal spice mixes and is indeed the basis for most Ayurvedic savories. I recommend tasting the spices individually first, to be sure you like them. If any flavor does not agree with you, you may reduce the amount of that spice and tailor the recipe to your own taste. (It's usually the fennel that takes some getting used to!)

1 tbsp whole coriander seed
1   tbsp whole cumin seed
1½ tsp whole fennel seed
1 tbsp turmeric powder

Dry roast the whole spices in a frying pan for a few minutes, just until they release their fragrance and you can smell them. Let them cool completely. In a coffee grinder reserved for spices or, alternatively, by hand with a mortar and pestle, grind to a uniform consistency. Transfer to a small mixing bowl and stir in the turmeric powder.

Using a teaspoon, a funnel, or a postcard folded in half to make a V-shaped chute, pour into a shaker jar with an airtight lid for storage.

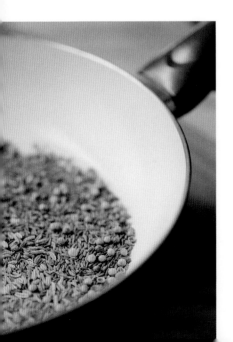

EVERYDAY SWEET SPICE MIX

makes ¼ cup

A must for cool mornings, this spice mix is the one to reach for whenever you want to add or enhance the sweet taste, and it offers a warming quality to aid digestion. There is no harm in using the Everyday Sweet Spice Mix generously, as there could be with sugar and other sweeteners. In fall and winter, you can turn most grain dishes into a breakfast with this mix; use it to add flavor to cooked fruits or add it to warm milk to make an instant spiced drink.

2 tbsp cinnamon powder

2 tbsp ginger powder

1 tbsp cardamom powder

Mix the powdered spices together in a glass shaker jar. Use anytime of year.

NOTE: In Ayurveda it is generally recommended to grind fresh, whole spices, but these three are not convenient to grind at home. I recommend buying them in powdered form, in small amounts from the bulk section at a store with good turnover to ensure freshness, or from a supplier in the "Resources" section (page 320).

EVERYDAY DIGESTIVE SALTS

makes ½ heaping cup

Salt, ginger, and lemon are known to increase the digestive fire by encouraging the correct ratio of fire and water in the stomach. Adding digestive salts to your meals instead of plain salt will get your digestive juices really flowing. Use salt moderately in the spring, when the water element accumulates, and in summer, when the fire element accumulates, as salt promotes both water and fire in the body.

1 dainty organic lemon
(Meyer if you can find one)

½ tsp fennel seeds (optional)

½ cup sea salt or pink salt

½ tsp ginger powder

Preheat oven to 300 degrees.

Make lemon zest by grating the outside of the lemon with a fine grater.

Grind the fennel seeds, if using, as fine as you can in a mortar and pestle or spices-only coffee grinder.

Mix 1 tsp lemon zest, the ground fennel seeds, salt, and ginger powder together in a bowl and spread the mixture out on a baking sheet, making sure there are no clumps. Bake for about 15 minutes, long enough to dry out the lemon zest. If the zest pieces look too large to pass through a shaker top, grind again with mortar and pestle.

Cool completely and transfer to a shaker jar.

everyday vegetable broth

makes 3½ cups

Vegetable broth can be enjoyed plain as a beverage with a meal, to replace a meal, or to tide you over between meals. Used as the base for soups and in cooking grains and beans, your broth enhances not only flavor but also nutrition. You can keep a bag of washed organic vegetable scraps (like celery tops, carrot peels, and sweet potato skins) in the freezer as you cook and once a week boil them with herbs or gingerroot to make your own fresh broth. Or you can start from scratch.

5 cups roughly chopped vegetables (carrots, potatoes, leeks, kale, parsnips, fennel) and/or vegetable skins

2 tbsp ghee

1 handful fresh herbs, stem included (thyme, rosemary, oregano, sage, parsley) or 2-inch piece fresh gingerroot, washed and thickly sliced

½ tsp salt

pinch of freshly ground black pepper

7 cups water

In a large, heavy-bottomed pot, sauté the vegetables in the ghee over medium heat until they begin to soften, about 10 minutes, stirring occasionally. Add the fresh herbs or gingerroot, salt, black pepper, and water and bring to a boil. Reduce heat to low, partially cover, and simmer 60 minutes. Remove from heat and strain through a fine mesh metal sieve into a glass bowl, saucepan, or other heatproof container, pressing on the vegetables with the back of a spoon to extract as much flavorful liquid as possible.

Allow broth to cool and then transfer to storage jars. Refrigerate for up to 1 week. If freezing, use within 1 month.

BROTH ALTERNATIVES

If you aren't finding the time to make your own broth, you can try using a concentrated vegetable paste, such as Better than Bouillon; organic bouillon cubes; or boxed premade broth. The ideal is to make your own, of course, and when I don't have any on hand, I tend to rely on the flavors of the Everyday spice mixes, quality salt, and the vegetables themselves in my recipes. If you do buy bouillon cubes and you are sensitive to wheat, look for ones that don't use wheat flour as a binder.

everyday ghee

makes 6 ounces

Otherwise known as clarified butter, often used in French cooking, ghee is considered to be the most beneficial cooking medium in Ayurveda and the jewel in the crown of Ayurvedic healing. This oil has the highest heat tolerance, is light enough to digest easily, and penetrates the body's tissues, providing the necessary nourishment and unsaturated fat to the deep tissue layers. Think of ghee as a carrier that brings the goods deep into the body. When spices are tempered in ghee, their medicinal qualities become available to these tissues. It must be of a medicinal quality, and so organic butter of the highest quality must be the base for this recipe.

To make ghee you remove the solids from the butter by cooking it over low heat. As it cooks, the water will be released in the form of tiny bubbles, and the solids will separate out, to be strained and discarded. The trick is not to let it burn, and so you must stay present with the butter for the full 15 minutes it takes to separate. Watch as it changes form and take great pride in every batch of golden yellow, spoonable cooking oil you create. Ghee making is a very satisfying and fun job that turns you into a kitchen healer.

This recipe makes roughly a 2-week supply. Once you get the hang of it you can double the recipe and make it monthly.

EXTRAS

½ lb (2 sticks) organic
unsalted butter

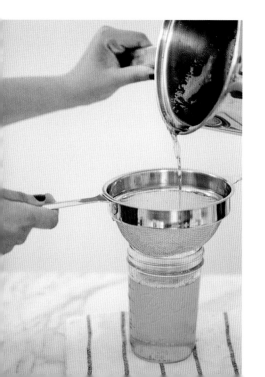

Place 2 sticks of butter in a small saucepan. Melt the butter over medium heat, then reduce the heat to low. After about 5 minutes the butter will begin to form a white froth on its surface, and you will hear popping sounds from the moisture evaporating. Continue to monitor the ghee; do not walk away or multitask. Notice when the popping sounds become more intermittent, and then it's time to hover. When the solids on the bottom of the pan begin to turn golden brown (after about 10–15 minutes), remove from heat.

Cool until it's just warm, for about 15 minutes. Strain through a strainer or cheesecloth into a sterilized glass jar (an empty nut butter jar works nicely). Skim off any last bits of foam that might remain.

Everyday Ghee does not need refrigeration for 1 month or so; keep it on the counter with a lid on, and always use a clean utensil when taking ghee from the jar. If you want to keep it longer, I recommend storing it in the fridge, but take it out to soften when you start cooking.

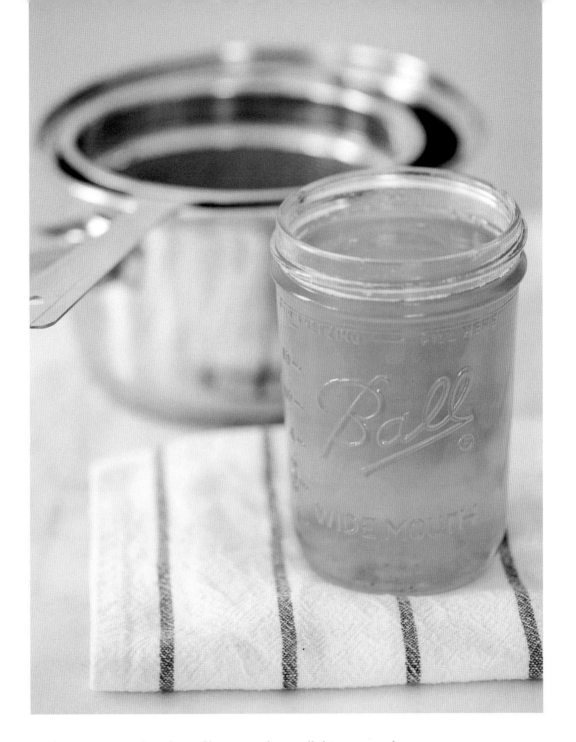

Ghee is great used in place of butter in almost all things: spread on toast, as a cooking oil for eggs, stirred into grains. It does have a different flavor and texture than butter and so will not integrate into finicky baking recipes, but you will certainly find it in my baked goods!

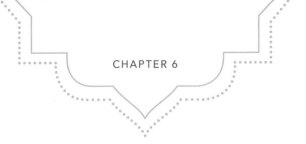

CHAPTER 6

Spring Recipes

WARM, LIGHT, WELL-SPICED MEALS TO BALANCE COOL, DAMP CLIMATES

The rivers are swollen with snowmelt, and the sap is starting to run in the trees. All the moisture that was bound by freezing temperatures is now moving to clear winter stagnation. And for our bodies, spring is the optimal time for lightening and clearing. Accumulated heavy and dense qualities from winter must be broken down and burned up. The body's need for the rich foods of winter shifts to a desire for light, dry, simple foods that digest easily. Stoke the digestive fires and encourage the body's natural cleansing this time of year with the pungent, bitter, and astringent tastes found in seasonal greens, bright berries, fresh ginger, turmeric, and spicy soups.

Spring Diet and Lifestyle Overview

The Elements: Earth and water
Feels Like: Heavy, cool, damp, slow, cloudy, sticky, stable

QUALITIES TO INTRODUCE/REDUCE

Introduce	*Reduce*
Warming	Cold
Light	Heavy
Dry	Oily
Mobile (get moving)	Static (sitting around)
Sharp	Dull
Penetrating	Slow

POTENTIAL SIGNS AND SYMPTOMS OF IMBALANCE

Loss of appetite

Sinus or chest congestion

Seasonal spring allergies

Lackluster or lethargic feelings

TASTES TO ENJOY

Bitter

Astringent

Pungent

Spring Foods Guide

Favor foods that are warm, light, and well spiced.

FOODS TO FAVOR

- Pungent spices, such as ginger, black pepper, lemon, and turmeric
- Dry grains, such as barley, rye, corn, millet, and buckwheat
- Astringent fruits, such as apples, pears, berries, dried cherries, raisins, and prunes. In cold climates, mostly dried fruits are available
- Lean proteins, such as beans, lentils, and egg whites; white meat for nonvegetarians
- Bitter vegetables, such as arugula, Brussels sprouts, cabbage, broccoli, dandelion greens, and asparagus
- Raw honey, in moderation

FOODS TO REDUCE

- Anything cold
- Dairy products

- Sweet, heavy fruits, such as dates, figs, and bananas
- Wheat
- Sweeteners (except raw honey)
- Fatty meats
- Roasted nuts
- Salt

SPRING LIFESTYLE GUIDELINES

- Use a light oil for massage (almond, grapeseed) and practice dry brushing a few times per week or daily, in the morning before your shower. You may add energizing natural scents to your massage oil, such as lemon, grapefruit, bergamot, pine, or tulsi oils.
- Practice neti (nasal irrigation) with a neti pot at morning shower time when the allergy season starts or before congestion begins to gather.
- Exercise daily, preferably first thing in the morning and outdoors, and make a point of getting a little sweaty.
- Take saunas.
- Reduce napping during the day and wake up with the sun.
- Do not eat when you're not hungry, and have a lighter breakfast than you were accustomed to in winter.
- Drink tulsi, ginger, or Spring Digestive Tea daily.

SPRING SHOPPING LIST

VEGETABLES	FRUITS	GRAINS	FATS	EXTRAS
Artichokes, fresh	Spinach	Amaranth	Tofu (served warm)	Red chilies, dried
Artichokes, marinated	Sprouts	Barley	White beans	Sambar powder
Arugula	Apples	Buckwheat		Star anise
Asparagus	Berries, fresh	Cornmeal (tortillas)	Goat cheese	Apple cider vinegar
Broccoli	Cherries, dried	Millet	Grapeseed oil	Balsamic vinegar
Cabbage	Cranberry juice	Rye	Hemp milk	Rice vinegar
Cauliflower	Grapefruit		Rice milk	Honey, raw
Daikon radish	Pears	BEANS	Soy milk	Natural bristle dry brush
Endive	Pomegranate juice	Black beans		
Fiddleheads	Prunes	Chickpeas	SPICES	
Leeks	Raisins	Green lentils	Fenugreek seeds	
Radicchio		Red lentils	Mustard seeds	

berry buck-up cereal

serves 2

I am always excited to come home from yoga and eat this cereal. Buckwheat is technically not a grain but a seed, and it is dry, slightly diuretic, and warming. Paired with the brightness of berries, it will help you "buck up" and get ready for the day. You will likely find it under the brand name Kashi, in its toasted form, which brings a roasted, nutty taste to this quick breakfast. Buckwheat is gluten free, easy on the blood sugar, and a good choice for mucus conditions, weight loss, and damp, cool weather. For a treat, top it with Berry Sweet Fruit Dip (see page 150).

(see page 150).

2 cups water

½ cup dry buckwheat, roasted or raw

1–2 tsp Everyday Sweet Spice Mix (see page 118)

½ tsp vanilla extract

1 cup chopped strawberries

2 tsp coconut oil

¼ cup shredded coconut

In a medium saucepan, bring 2 cups water to a boil. Rinse the buckwheat in a strainer and add the buckwheat, the spice mix, and the vanilla to the boiling water. Turn heat to low, cover, and simmer for 15 minutes. Remove from heat, add strawberries and coconut oil, and fluff with a fork. Cover again and let stand for 5 minutes.

While buckwheat is resting, toast the shredded coconut in a small frying pan over low heat for a few minutes, stirring constantly, until it begins to brown.

To serve, divide the buckwheat into two bowls and sprinkle toasted coconut on top.

HINT: if you soak the buckwheat overnight, it will cook in 10 minutes. You can soak the coconut as well to soften its texture and produce a creamier cereal. If you do, skip the step for toasting coconut.

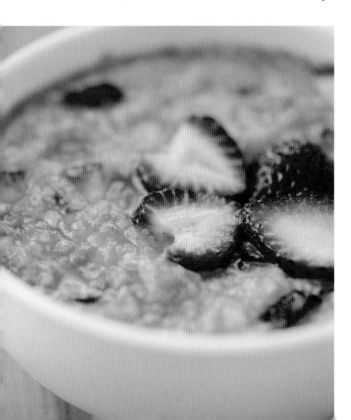

cherry millet cakes

makes 6

Millet is a dry, chewy grain, a good choice for damp weather. These cakes call on the astringency of cherries and prunes and the warmth of fresh ginger to support the body in getting rid of excess damp and cool qualities. A Cherry Millet Cake is a good replacement for white flour- and white sugar-based pastries, which can really gum up the works as the body clears out winter stagnation. If you think you might crave a pastry later, pack one or two of these.

⅓ cup prunes

1 cup cooked millet

1 tbsp ground flaxseed

½ tsp ginger powder

1 tsp lemon juice

¼ cup dried cherries

1 tbsp uncooked millet grains

Preheat oven to 400 degrees. Line muffin tins with 6 baking cups. In a medium mixing bowl, soak the prunes in ⅓ cup warm water for 15 minutes. Using a hand blender, puree the prunes and their soaking liquid with ¼ cup of the cooked millet. Stir together the prune and millet puree, ground flaxseed, ginger powder, and lemon juice. Add the remaining ¾ cup of cooked millet and the cherries and stir to combine. Let rest 5 minutes.

Evenly divide the mixture among the muffin cups, sprinkle with uncooked millet, and gently press each millet cup with the back of a spoon to smooth the top. Bake 20–25 minutes, until firm and browned on top.

ONLY RAW HONEY

Raw honey is the preferred springtime sweetener because of its warming, cleansing qualities. However, the Ayurvedic texts caution against the heating of honey during cooking. Conventional honey has been cooked during processing, which renders it an indigestible, sticky substance that ends up in the body as ama, or toxicity. If you need more sweet taste than you are getting from the spring recipes, smear a teaspoon of raw honey on your treats before serving—but do not bake with it. If you are adding it to tea, make sure the water is not boiling hot—let it cool one minute before stirring in honey.

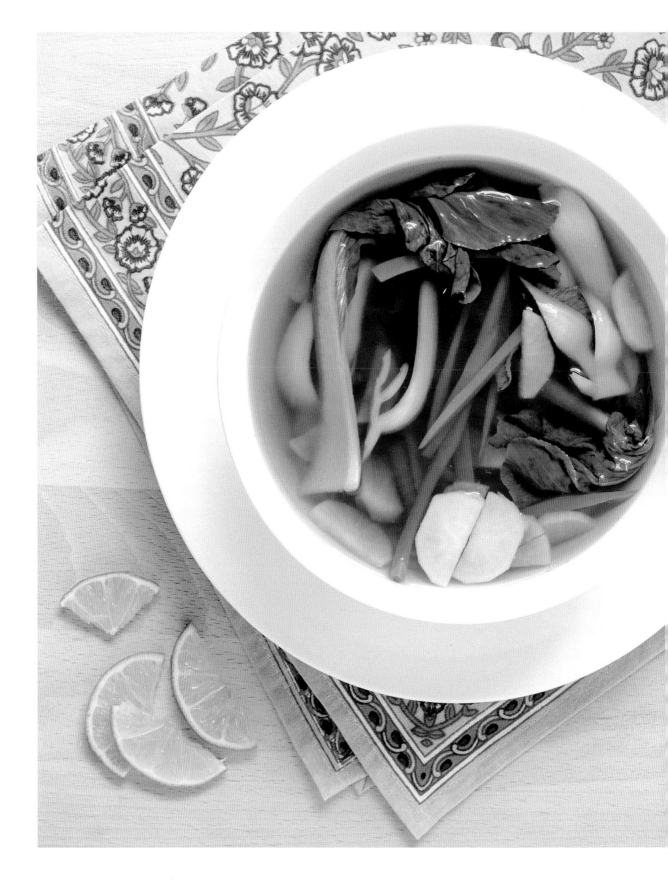

savory breakfast soup

serves 2

This recipe is an adaptation of a traditional southern Vietnamese breakfast. The pungency of savory, slightly spicy tastes for breakfast (instead of sweet and cool, such as we get with cold cereals) will stoke the digestive fires during a damp season, when they tend to run low. In line with Ayurvedic principles, in the warm southern region of Vietnam, breakfast pho soup has a sweet broth and is seasoned with fresh herbs, which are cooling. In the cool northern regions, the soup more often contains vinegar and chili, which are heating. This version falls on the milder side of what you might find in pho's homeland, but I make up for the mildness by adding fresh ginger.

4   cups water

1   medium carrot

2   stalks bok choy or 1 head
    baby bok choy

1   daikon radish, about 6
    inches long

2   tsp freshly grated ginger

black pepper to taste

1   tbsp tamari

1   small lime, juiced

lime wedges for garnish

OPTIONAL ADDITIONS

1   large handful Zucchini
    Noodles (see page 186) or
    rice noodles; replace 1 cup
    water with 1 cup coconut milk

Boil the water in a large saucepan. Coarsely chop the vegetables and add to the pan. Add freshly grated ginger and black pepper to taste and simmer, covered, for 5 minutes. If using zucchini or rice noodles, add for the last minute of cooking and cover again. Simmer until vegetables and noodles are al dente. Take off the heat and add lime juice and tamari.

To serve, ladle soup into 2 wide noodle bowls. Accompany with fresh lime wedges.

south indian sambar

serves 4

Sambar, a tomato, dal, and tamarind soup served with rice, is a staple of south Indian cuisine, eaten for breakfast as well as lunch. On my first trip to south India, spicy sambar for breakfast took some getting used to. It was everywhere, all the time, and I could never be quite sure what those floating vegetables were. Years later, I don't feel I have arrived in the south until I've had a cup of authentic sambar, and I make it often at home in winter and spring. To keep it very simple for you, I have veered from tradition a bit here by using premade sambar powder that you can buy from an Indian grocer and only ingredients you can find easily. This is a great spring recipe because of its hot, light, pungent, and sour qualities. If your stomach gets aggravated by spicy or sour food, reduce the sambar powder to make it less spicy and reduce the tomato to make it less sour.

4 cups water

½ cup yellow split mung beans, rinsed twice

1 tsp turmeric

2 small tomatoes, coarsely chopped

½ cup coarsely chopped carrot

½ cup coarsely chopped green bean

½ cup coarsely chopped daikon radish

1 tbsp coconut oil

1 small onion, diced (optional)

1 tsp mustard seeds

2 sprigs fresh curry leaf (optional)

2 pinches hing (asafetida)

¼ cup grated coconut (see sidebar)

1–2 tsp sambar powder

salt to taste

fresh cilantro for garnish (optional)

Bring the water to a boil in a large saucepan. Add the mung beans and turmeric powder and bring to a boil again. Add the chopped vegetables to the pot, except onion, if using. Turn heat down to low and simmer, partially covered for 30 minutes.

While the dal is cooking, heat the coconut oil in a frying pan and fry the diced onion on medium heat until translucent, about 5 minutes. Stir in the mustard seeds; these will splutter, so cover before frying for 1 minute. Add curry leaf and stir, then add hing and stir until all the spices are coated with the oil. When you can smell the spices, turn off the heat. Stir the grated coconut into the hot oil mixture and let stand for 1-2 minutes.

Add the spiced oil and sambar powder to the cooked dal in the saucepan. Simmer all together for 5 minutes, adding hot water if the sambar is getting too thick—it should be a bit watery. Add salt to taste.

Serve in 4 bowls with Everyday Dosa or pour over basmati rice. Garnish with fresh cilantro, if you like. Adventure-chef note: for a more authentic and sour flavor, you may also stir in 2-3 tsp of tamarind paste when you add the tomato.

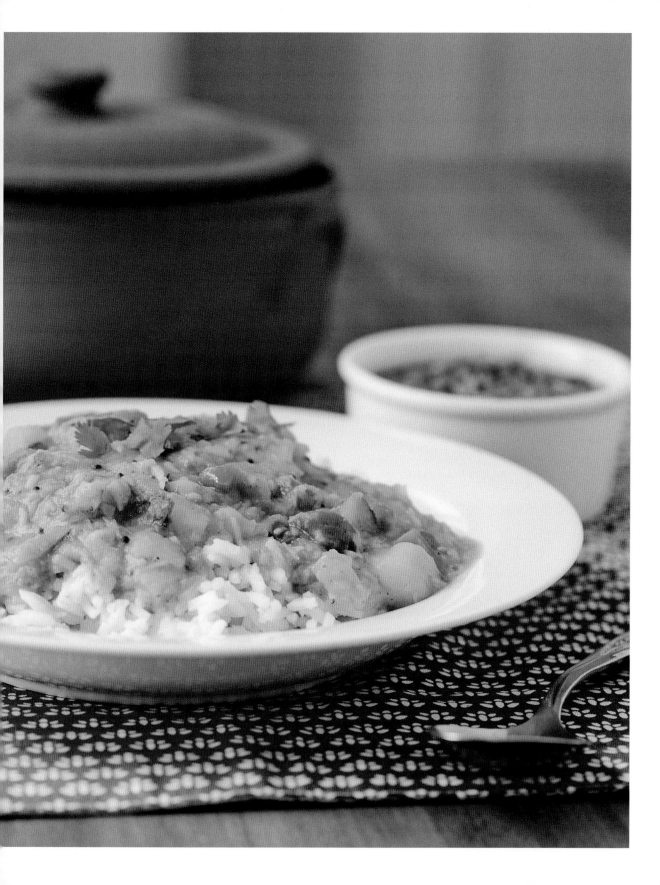

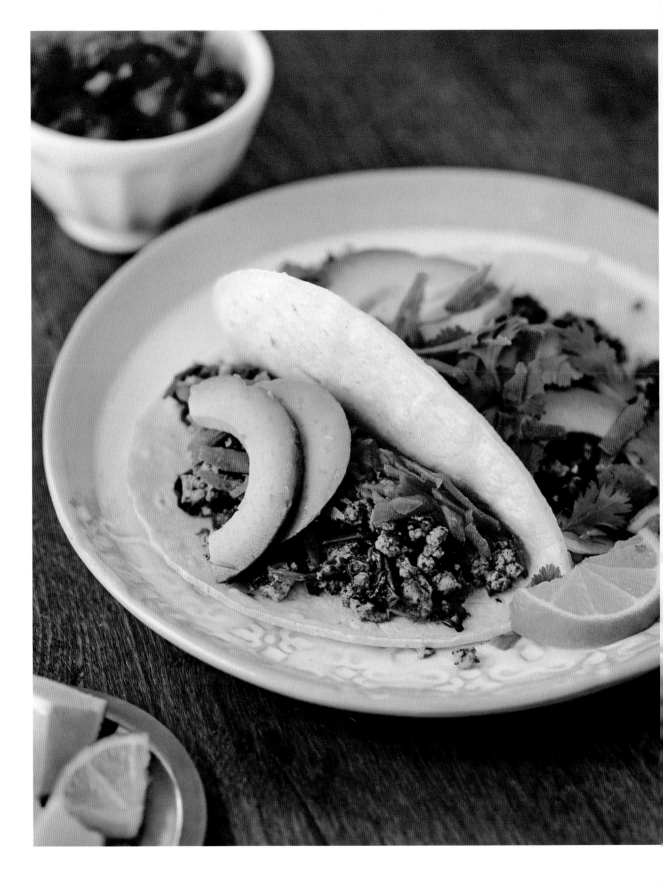

tofu tacos with greens

serves 2

On a cold, dry spring day you may have a heartier appetite than on a warm, wet day. Tofu Tacos with Greens make an easy, satisfying meal for a hearty day while staying aligned with the lighter qualities of spring. The dry quality of corn, the bitter taste of the greens, and a hint of spice to help the body digest tofu's proteins balance the meal so you will feel full, but not heavy. Raw Beet Slaw with Lemon and Mint (see page 224) makes a great side dish for these tacos—just omit the mint and sunflower seeds to keep the flavors simple.

1 tsp chili powder

½ tsp cumin powder

½ tsp coriander powder

½ tsp turmeric powder

pinch of black pepper or cayenne pepper

¼ tsp salt

½ 14-oz block of extra firm tofu

2 tsp sunflower oil or ghee

1 cup roughly chopped baby spinach or Swiss chard

4 corn tortillas

½ lime, cut into wedges

TOPPINGS, IN ANY COMBINATION:

fresh salsa

sliced avocados

chopped cilantro

shredded carrots

shredded lettuce

Combine all the spices and the salt in a small mixing bowl.

Rinse the tofu well and squeeze it between your palms to remove some of the water. This will make it cook faster. In a small bowl, mash the tofu with a fork, then stir into the spice mixture.

In a medium frying pan, warm the oil or ghee on medium-low heat. When the pan is hot, add the tofu and fry, using a spatula to stir well every few minutes. After 5 minutes, add the chopped greens and fold in with the spatula. Continue cooking and stirring for 5 minutes more. When the tofu begins to brown, remove from heat and cover to keep warm.

Pat each tortilla with damp hands to soften. In another large frying pan, spread the tortillas in a single layer and warm over low heat for 2-3 minutes. If the edges begin to curl, take them off the heat immediately.

To serve, place 2 tortillas side by side on 2 plates and spoon a strip of tofu mixture on each tortilla. Add toppings in any combination. Accompany with fresh lime wedges to squeeze on top. Fold in half to eat as soft tacos.

NOTE: If your body doesn't digest tofu well, substitute 4-6 egg whites, lightly scrambled.

If you are a fan of garlic and onion, spring is a good time of year to eat them, in moderation. Most people who don't experience signs of acid stomach can enjoy a small amount of either food, well cooked, twice a week or so. Fry 2 tbsp chopped red onion and ½ clove peeled, chopped garlic for 5 minutes, then stir in the tofu and continue frying. Go easy on the fresh salsa, as it usually contains raw onion and garlic.

asparagus and white bean soup

serves 2

I created this recipe by making Everyday Cream of Anything Soup (see page 92) as a base and adding the lemony Spring Salts. It is such a simple and delicious way to eat asparagus that this soup earned a spot in my core spring recipes. Eating asparagus in springtime, when the stalks are small and tender, is a real joy, and the vegetable purifies the body's water element. The recipe has a reduced amount of oil to help your body manage the damp quality of springtime.

1 bunch asparagus stalks
2 cups water
1 tsp olive oil
½ cup cooked white beans
1 tsp Spring Salts
juice of ¼ lemon
¼ lemon cut into 2 wedges
freshly ground black pepper
    to taste

Chop about 1–2 inches off the bottom of the asparagus stalks to remove the woody part. Chop the stalks into 1-inch pieces. In a medium saucepan, boil the asparagus with 1 cup of the water until the asparagus is tender, about 7 minutes. Put the asparagus and cooking water in a blender carafe along with the other cup of water, olive oil, beans, and Spring Salts and blend on medium-high until smooth. (Or put the additional ingredients right in the pot, turn off the heat, and process with an immersion hand blender.) Put the soup back in the saucepan and warm on low heat until hot enough to serve. Remove from heat and stir in juice of ¼ lemon.

Serve in 2 bowls, with lemon wedges and freshly ground black pepper.

NOTE: Broccoli is a nice substitute for asparagus and offers the same light qualities of bitter taste. If you are new to the Ayurvedic diet, I think you will take comfort in the familiarity of an old standby like cream of broccoli soup.

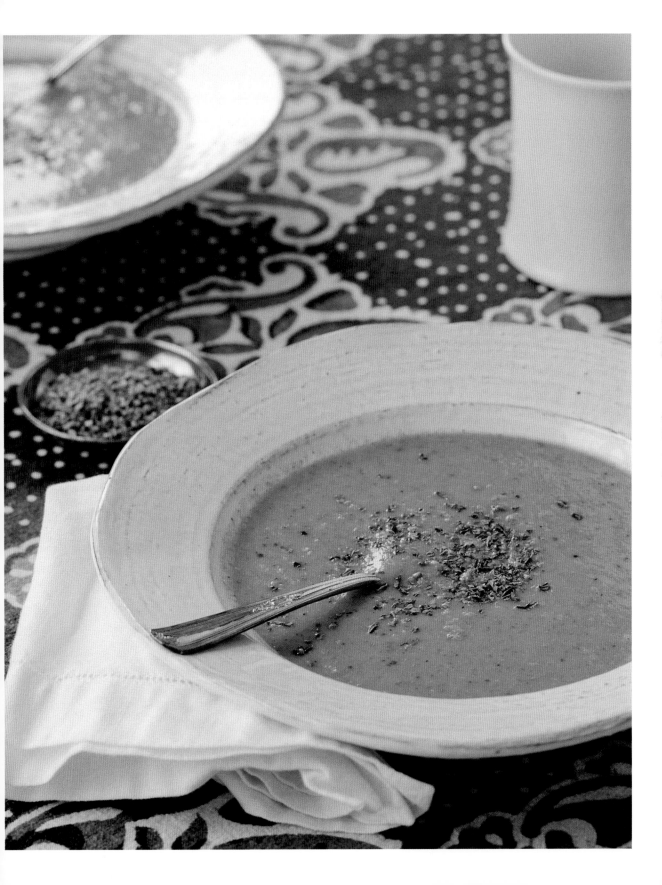

spicy andhra-style dal

serves 4

Spring is the best time of year to enjoy the pungent taste, such as one finds in mustard seeds, chilies, and garlic. This dal reflects the cookery of the south Indian state Andhra Pradesh, home of favorite *thali* (lunch) and India's leading producer of red chilies. The tangy, spicy nature of this dish, along with the light, dry qualities of whole mung beans and the added fiber of the bean's skin, makes for a cleansing meal when the weather is damp and cool.

1 cup whole green mung beans

1 tbsp ghee

1 big or 3 small dried
   red chilies

1-inch piece fresh gingerroot,
   peeled and grated

½ tbsp Spring Spice Mix (see
   page 158)

2 tsp mustard seeds

2 tsp cumin seeds

4 cups water

juice of 1 lemon

½ tsp salt

Soak the mung beans in water overnight or use the quick-soak method (see page 303). When ready to cook, drain and rinse the soaked mung beans.

Heat the ghee over medium heat in a large pot. Add the chilies, grated ginger, spice mix, and the mustard and cumin seeds. Stir until the mustard seeds begin to pop, a few minutes. Add the mung beans to the pot and stir until the ghee and spices are evenly distributed. Add the water, partially cover the pot, and boil for 30 minutes, or until the beans begin to break up. Keep an eye on the water level, as you may need to add a bit of hot water during cooking if the dal becomes dry. When the beans are completely soft, remove from heat and add the lemon juice and salt.

Serve in a wide bowl or plate, over basmati rice.

MUSTARD SEEDS HAVE A MIND OF THEIR OWN

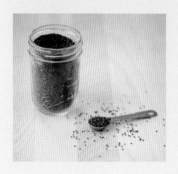

I feel I should warn you about frying mustard seeds. It has taken me some time to figure this out, but I always keep a lid nearby for the frying pan. As the mustard seeds begin to cook, they will pop and can bounce out of the pan like popcorn. To allow them to fry for 1 minute while they are rebelling, cover loosely. Then be quick about it as you pull off the cover to add the next ingredients. Those mustard seeds will settle right down.

simple stovetop tofu

serves 2-3

Anyone living in a vegetarian household knows about tofu's high-protein versatility. This recipe is often requested for yoga potlucks—and is easy to double or triple. Coated with cheesy-tasting nutritional yeast, this tofu has long been a favorite supper of mine, which meant it had to be included in this book. Excellent served atop a pile of steamed kale.

1 12-oz block extra firm tofu
2 tbsp ghee
2 tbsp nutritional yeast
2 tbsp tamari

Drain and rinse the tofu. Press gently to squeeze out excess water. Cut the tofu into 1-inch cubes.

Melt the ghee in a large frying pan over medium-low heat. Place the tofu cubes in a single layer in the pan. Fry for about 7 minutes, or until lightly browned. You may need to gently shake the pan every few minutes to keep the tofu from sticking. Then flip the cubes over with a spatula.

When the other sides are browned and all liquid is gone, another 7 minutes or so, remove from the heat. While the tofu is still in the frying pan, sprinkle it with the nutritional yeast, then the tamari. Stir with the spatula to coat the cubes, adding more yeast or tamari if needed to achieve the desired "cheesiness."

Serve warm tofu cubes on top of an Everyday Steamed Salad Bowl or greens.

WHAT IS NUTRITIONAL YEAST?

Nutritional yeast is found in the supplement section at health food stores. It is not a traditional Ayurvedic ingredient, but its qualities in the Ayurvedic spectrum are light and dry. This food-based supplement (i.e. not made of synthetic, chemical ingredients) provides protein and a cheesy taste and feel without the heavy, oily qualities of dairy cheese. The yeast is not active, as is baker's yeast, and therefore does not expand in the belly. Nutritional yeast is not like brewer's yeast, either, a high-protein by-product of the brewing process. It is grown primarily to be used as a supplement. The live yeast predigests B vitamins, rendering them easily absorbed by the body. Heating the yeast reduces the efficacy of the vitamins. Nutritional yeast is a good source of protein and amino acids, which vegetarian diets sometimes lack. This powder can also thicken a soup and make it taste cheesy.

Unless you just want to buy a little to see if you like it, it is best not to buy nutritional yeast from the bulk bins, as it has oxidized. When it is fresh it has a bright yellow color, which fades as it ages. Buy it prepackaged in a sealed canister, which keeps it at its most fresh.

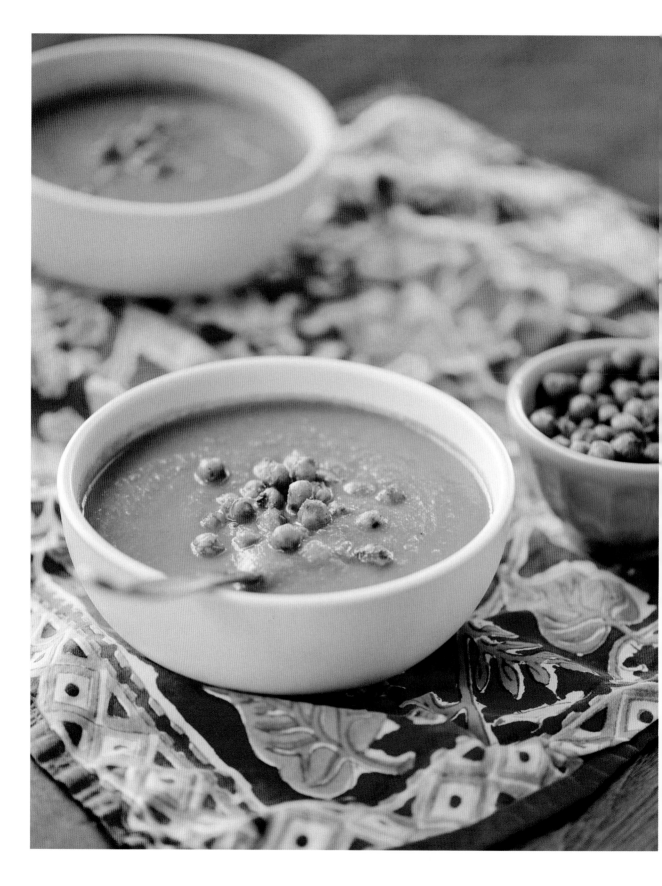

carrot ginger soup with roasted chickpeas

serves 4

Sweet and spicy: you can't go wrong with this soup, which is beneficial for anybody, anytime and a simple way to boost your spring ginger intake. Once you know how to make Carrot Ginger Soup, you will want to get in the habit of having it often. Carrots have a relaxing, cooling effect on the eyes, so consider making this soup when you are spending a lot of time in front of the computer screen. A garnish of Roasted Chickpeas adds texture and crunch, as well as the beneficial dry quality of beans.

4 cups water

2 tsp coriander powder

1 lb carrots

2–3 inches fresh gingerroot

2 tsp ghee, olive oil, or sunflower oil, plus 2 tsp more for drizzling

dash each of salt and pepper

Roasted Chickpeas

In a medium saucepan, begin to boil 4 cups water and coriander powder. Coarsely chop the carrots and add to the pot. Peel and roughly dice the gingerroot and add to the pot. Boil for 15–20 minutes, covered, until carrots are tender. Add ghee or oil, salt, and pepper. With an immersion hand blender, blend until smooth, or transfer to a carafe blender and cool for 2–3 minutes before blending on low, then high until smooth.

Ladle into 4 soup bowls, topping each serving with ¼ cup Roasted Chickpeas and ½ tsp ghee or oil.

ROASTED CHICKPEAS

serves 6-8

Behold the chickpea: high in protein, high in flavor, low in fat. Chickpeas are popular in all regions of India, and roasted chickpeas served in newspaper cones are a common street food, like the paper bags of peanuts Americans enjoy at baseball games. This a great spring garnish, on the dry and spicy side. Try Roasted Chickpeas atop soup or on an Everyday Steamed Salad Bowl. Better not to eat them on their own when you are very hungry, because too much dry food will slow down your digestion. As with all foods dry and crunchy, use moderation.

2 cups cooked chickpeas

2 tbsp apple cider vinegar

2 tsp Spring Spice Mix (see page 158)

1 tsp cumin powder

dash of salt

2 tsp sunflower oil

Preheat oven to 400 degrees.

Rinse and drain the chickpeas well. Wrap them in a clean towel and shake them to get some water off, then place them in a large bowl. Sprinkle the vinegar, spices, salt, and oil over them. Mix together with your hands, rubbing the savory ingredients well into the chickpeas.

Spread the chickpeas on a baking sheet and bake for 40 minutes, stirring every 15 minutes. When the chickpeas are lightly browned, remove from the oven. (If you prefer them crunchy, bake for up to 50 minutes—but don't forget to stir, and watch to make sure they don't blacken.) Allow them to cool before storing in an airtight container at room temperature.

Alternatively, Roasted Chickpeas are also wonderful hot out of the oven, used as a garnish. This recipe will yield one extra cup to be stored after garnishing Carrot Ginger Soup.

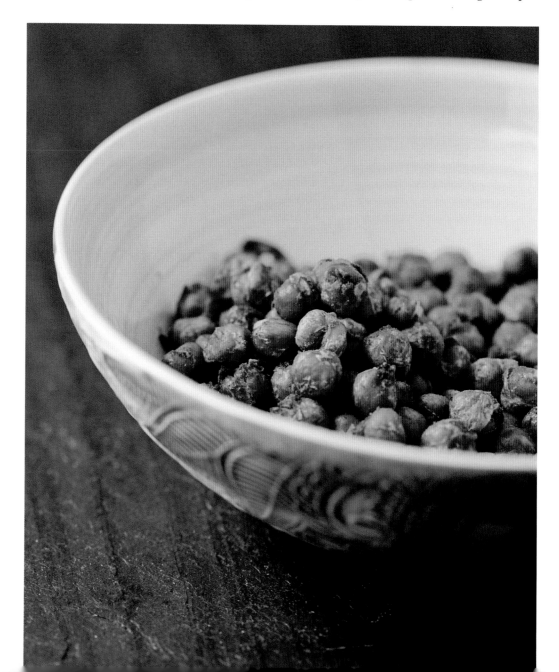

cauliflower leek soup

serves 2

Cauliflower replaces the potatoes of potato-leek soup recipes to create a light, yet creamy, seasonal soup. Your palate will not miss the potatoes, and your body will not miss the simple carbohydrates this time of year. Garnish with crunchy Roasted Chickpeas (see page 141) or serve with Easy Chana Dosa (see page 180) for more protein.

2 tsp sunflower or safflower oil
1 small head cauliflower
1 leek
4 cups broth
1 tsp Spring Salts

Warm the oil in a large saucepan over medium heat. While it is warming, chop the white part of the leek into thin 1-inch strips, and dice the cauliflower head into 1-inch pieces. Sauté the leek in the oil for 5 minutes, until soft. Add cauliflower, broth, and salts to the saucepan and simmer, covered, for 20 minutes, until cauliflower is soft. Remove from heat and puree the soup, right in the saucepan, with an immersion hand blender until smooth. For carafe blenders, transfer the contents of the saucepan into the carafe and cool for 2–3 minutes. Begin blending on low and increase speed until smooth.

Transfer to 2 large soup bowls for serving.

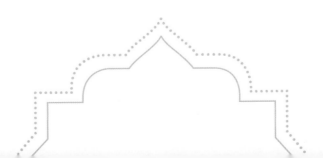

white bean and artichoke croquettes

makes 6

These light, lemony patties are nicely complemented by stone-ground mustard, which is helpful in springtime because its pungent taste is warming. Serve 2 croquettes on a bed of spring grains or alongside an Everyday Steamed Salad Bowl. These are a good option to pack for lunch, as they travel well.

SUPPER

1 cup cooked white cannellini beans

handful of baby spinach

2 marinated, drained artichoke hearts or 2 steamed artichoke hearts plus 1 tsp olive oil

1 tbsp ground flaxseed

1 tsp Spring Salts

¼ tsp lemon zest (optional)

Preheat the oven to 350 degrees. Line a baking sheet with parchment paper. In a large mixing bowl, mash the beans well with a fork. Chop the spinach and dice the artichoke, then stir the veggies into the mashed beans with the fork. Add the flaxseed, Spring Salts, lemon zest, and olive oil, if using steamed artichokes, as marinated will already contain oil. Stir until the mixture is a uniformly chunky consistency.

Form 6 patties, distribute on the parchment-paper-covered sheet, and bake for 10 minutes on each side. Alternatively, you can melt 1 tsp of ghee in a ceramic nonstick frying pan and pan fry the patties slowly over medium heat until browned, about 5 minutes for each side.

Serve with stone-ground mustard.

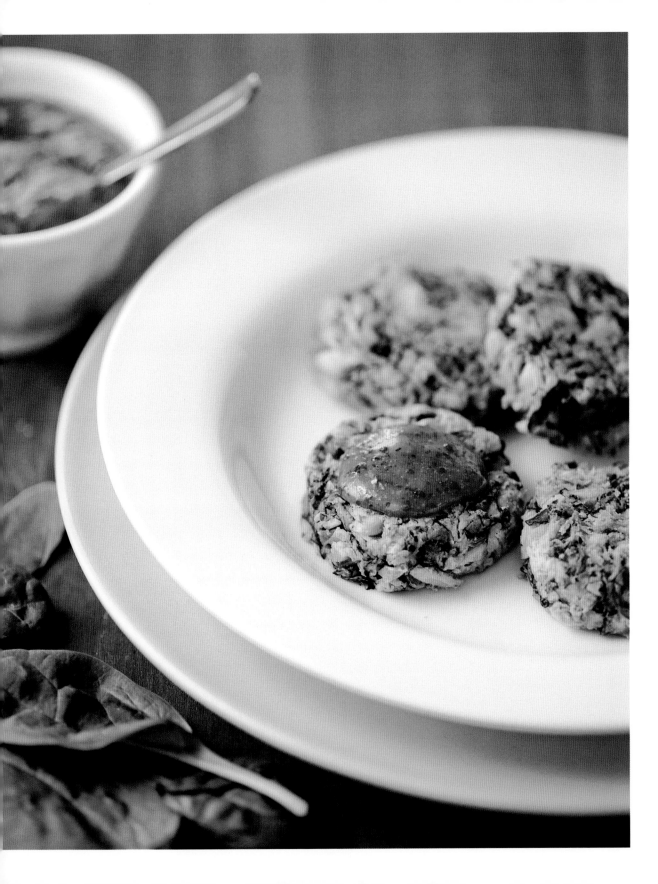

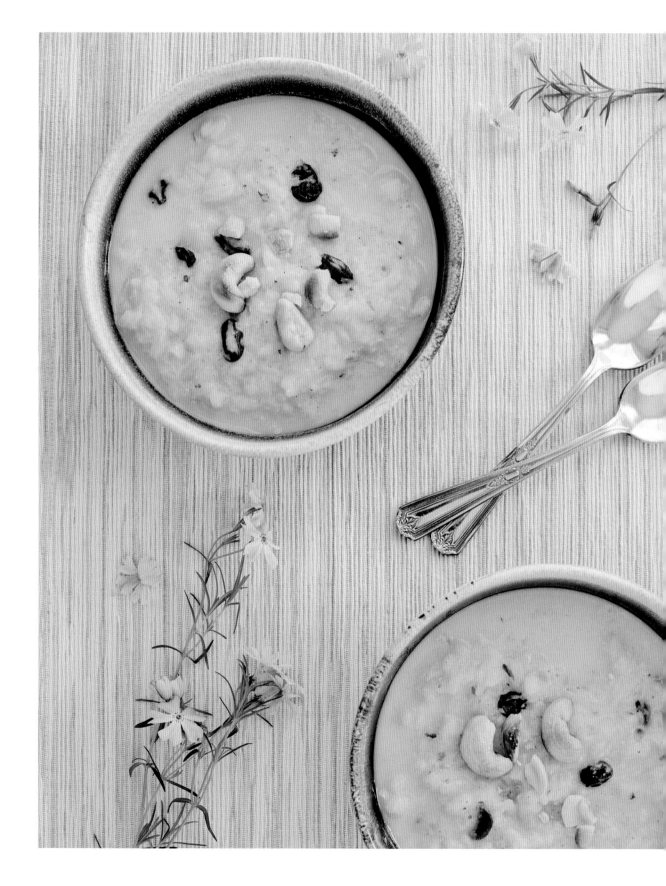

kheer light

serves 2

This rice pudding is a great way to use up extra rice left over from dinner for a dessert. Although the texture of traditional kheer is deeply rich and satisfying, the amount of milk and sugar usually used provide more building qualities than you need in spring. This version takes only about 20 minutes to prepare and contains light, warming qualities that are balancing for the springtime.

1 cup cooked white
    basmati rice
1¾ cup Everyday Almond Milk
    (see page 114)
1 tsp pure vanilla extract
2 tbsp raisins
10 soaked almonds, ground
    in coffee grinder or blender,
    or 1 tbsp almond flour
¼ tsp powdered cardamom
1 tsp freshly grated ginger
pinch of saffron thread
    (optional)
1 tsp raw honey (optional)

Warm the rice, almond milk, and vanilla extract together in a small pot over medium heat. Add the raisins, ground almonds or almond flour, cardamom, grated ginger, and saffron thread, if using. If you want to keep it simple, use the Everyday Sweet Spice Mix (see page 118) instead of the separate spices. Partially cover the pot, with the lid slightly ajar, and simmer on low heat for 15 minutes.

To serve, divide between 2 bowls. Stir ½ tsp honey into each serving, if desired.

NOTE: To make this rice pudding richer, use uncooked rice. Coarsely grind ½ cup raw basmati rice in a coffee grinder or blender, then simmer it in 1½ cups Everyday Almond Milk along with the other ingredients above for 1 hour. If you are trying to impress a guest, in a small frying pan toast 6 raw cashews in 1 tsp of ghee on the stovetop and garnish each pudding bowl with 3 golden cashews.

ON MODERATION

Ayurvedic meals often feature small amounts of ingredients that could be aggravating in larger quantities. Rather than omitting an ingredient, dishes will have just a sprinkle of roasted nuts, chopped chili, or potato, for example—enough to please the senses without accumulating in your system.

At an Ayurveda clinic on a local holiday, a reveler wandered in from the street with sweets to share. I was observing a cleansing diet that week, and when the man put a sweet in my hand that I "shouldn't" eat, I wanted to cry. Seeing my reaction, the doctor broke off a chunk and said, "Enjoy this small piece and be happy." This challenge to my "all or nothing" approach was the first step of a continuing path toward moderation and a true, mindful enjoyment of food.

notella hazelnut spread

makes 16 ounces

This version of a heating, oily chocolate spread takes care to keep it light by incorporating almonds and coconut milk instead of processed fats and whole milk powder. Soaking and skinning the almonds first makes this spread easier to digest and metabolize. The labor-intensive nut skinning will keep you from eating it too fast! Notella Hazelnut Spread is extremely satisfying on a piece of sprouted grain toast, when you get a hankering. Easy now, especially in springtime: a serving size is just 1 tablespoon.

¾ cup raw almonds
¾ cup raw hazelnuts
½ cup finely ground cacao powder
½ cup coconut milk
½ cup coconut sugar
1 tsp pure vanilla extract
pinch of salt

Soak the raw almonds 6–8 hours.

Preheat the oven to 350 degrees. Spread the soaked almonds and raw hazelnuts in a large baking pan and bake for 10 minutes, shaking the pan a few times. While they are still warm, wrap the nuts in a slightly damp kitchen towel. Rub the nuts between your palms to loosen and remove the skins. (A little bit of skin stuck on some won't hurt the final product.)

In a food processor, process the nuts until they are a uniform powder. Add the rest of the ingredients and process again until smooth and buttery.

Transfer to a 16-ounce glass jar and store in the refrigerator.

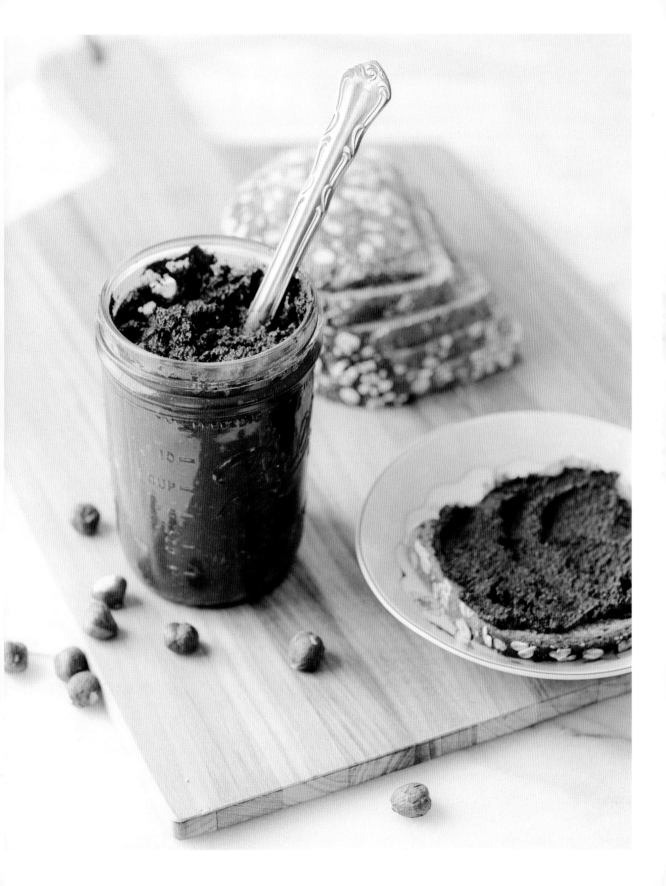

berry sweet fruit dip

serves 2

Spring is not the time to indulge a sweet tooth. Luckily the sweetness of early spring berries is balanced by their sharp, astringent qualities, which have a cleansing effect on the body. Because fruit digests at a faster rate than other foods, the optimal way to use this sauce is as a dip or spread with other fruits. Whip up Berry Sweet Fruit Dip quickly if you need a hit of sweetness, rather than reaching for artificial sugary stuff.

TREATS

2 tbsp golden raisins

2 tbsp apple or cherry juice

1 cup raspberries or blackberries

1 tsp Sweet Spice Mix (see page 118)

squeeze of fresh lemon, to taste

In a small mixing bowl, soak the raisins in the juice for about 10 minutes. Transfer the raisins and juice to a blender carafe (if using a regular blender) or a medium-sized bowl (if using a hand blender). Add the berries, spice mix, and fresh lemon juice and puree until smooth.

Serve in a cute bowl alongside sliced apples or pears.

KITCHEN CLOSED

Eating too much is a common reason the digestion and metabolism slow down and begin to have difficulty processing otherwise unproblematic foods. Suzanne was always trying to lose a little weight. But after a long day, she had difficulty putting aside half of the food she'd made that day; she'd eat it rather than saving it for tomorrow's lunch. She had a tendency to eat too fast and was also in the habit of eating with the TV on. I suggested she try eating while listening to mellow music, instead of the TV, and that she take a short walk outside soon after eating. When she slowed down the pace of her eating, she found it was easier to notice when she was full. If she still had a desire to eat more food or have dessert, she would put on a jacket and walk outside for just 15 minutes. The change of scenery and getting out of the kitchen were enough to shift her attention away from food cravings, and she could come back inside, clean up, and close the kitchen for the night.

ginger lime lassi

serves 2

Dairy is best diluted in springtime, if not avoided altogether. But a lassi with the light and penetrating qualities of ginger and honey renders a small amount of whole milk yogurt highly beneficial as a postmeal digestive. Be sure to use room temperature water, not cold.

¼ cup organic whole milk yogurt

1 cup water, room temperature

1-inch piece fresh gingerroot, peeled and coarsely chopped

juice of ½ small lime

1 tsp raw honey (optional)

Using a hand blender or carafe blender, churn together the yogurt, water, fresh ginger, lime juice, and honey, if using, on high speed for 1-2 minutes.

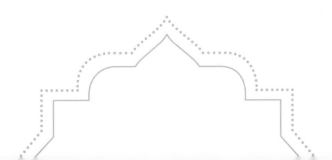

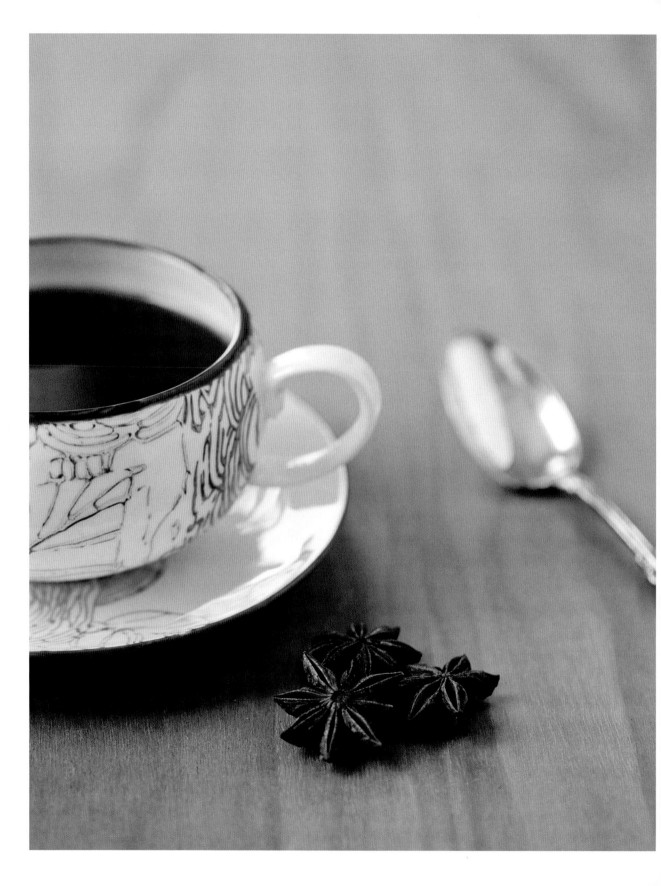

spring digestive tea

serves 2

This tea will warm up the belly and kick sluggish digestion lingering from winter into gear. To help you reduce sweets, which are not indicated this time of year, cinnamon also eases a sweet tooth and balances blood sugar.

. . . . ●●●●●● . . . .

2 cups water

½-inch piece fresh gingerroot

½ star anise

2–3 cloves

2–3 black peppercorns

½ tsp cinnamon powder

In a small saucepan bring 2 cups of water to a boil. Coarsely chop the gingerroot, including the skin. Add the chopped ginger, star anise, cloves, peppercorns, and cinnamon to the water. Reduce heat to low and simmer 10 minutes or longer. Strain into 2 mugs.

Drink 6 ounces with or after meals.

NOTE: Not everyone enjoys the taste of clove or anise. Nibble a corner of the whole spice to make sure the taste does not bother you before making this tea for the first time. If you experience acid indigestion at times, omit the black pepper. If you have a head or chest cold, add ½ tsp cumin seed to the recipe.

refresh-o-rama

serves 2

The penetrating quality of this bright drink clears your head and gets you pumped up without caffeine. Those who experience congestion upon waking will especially benefit from Refresh-O-Rama. It's best first thing in the morning, on an empty stomach. Wait at least 30 minutes before eating. If you find the drink too acidic, use lime instead of lemon juice and omit the cayenne pepper.

juice of 2 oranges or grapefruits
(about 2 cups juice)
1 ½-inch piece gingerroot,
peeled
1–2 tsp raw honey
juice of 1 lemon
dash of cayenne pepper for
the adventurous

Process 1 cup of the orange or grapefruit juice and the gingerroot in a blender until well combined. Keeping the blender running, drizzle the honey through the feeder, then pour in the rest of the orange or grapefruit juice, the lemon juice, and the cayenne pepper, if using. Churn for 1 minute.

Transfer to 2 glasses and drink right away, before the spices and pulp settle.

NOTE: I am not always in the mood for juicing, and then I peel the fruits, section them, pull out any seeds, and add all ingredients at once, blending to a smoothie consistency.

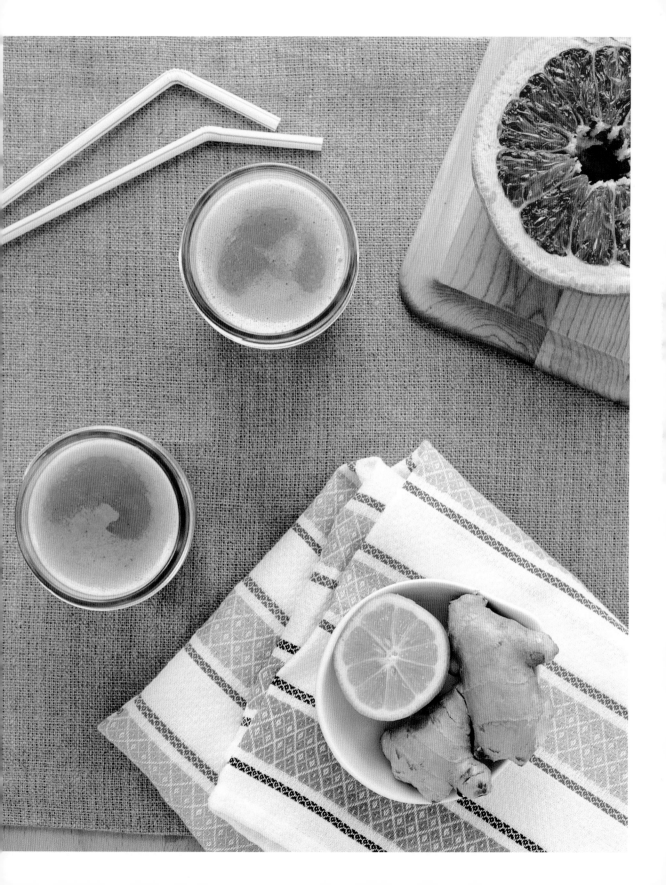

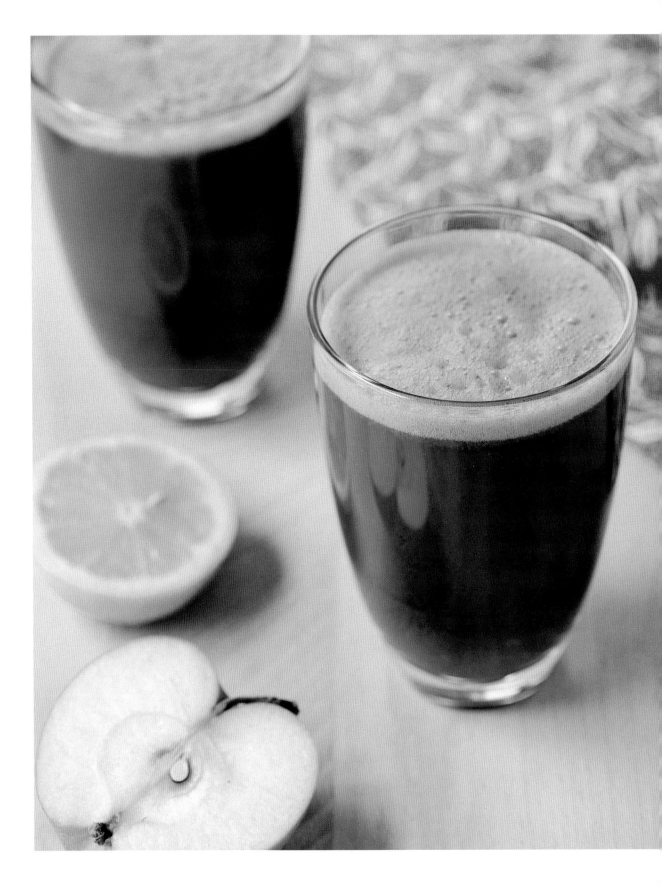

cleansing green juice

serves 2

This is an extremely cleansing beverage that kills cravings and makes a powerful snack. Sweet, slightly sour, bitter, and pungent tastes meld into a balanced juice that can be made with or without a juicer.

2   apples, cored and cut into quarters

4   kale leaves or 2 handfuls baby spinach

juice of 1 lemon

1-inch piece fresh ginger, peeled and roughly chopped

Combine all ingredients in a blender carafe with 1½ cups water. Blend until it reaches a smooth juice consistency (more watery than a smoothie), adding more water if desired or necessary.

To serve, strain the mixture through a large strainer into 2 glasses, pushing the juice through with the back of a spoon.

spring ayurvedic spice mix and salts

Most spring recipes call for a bit of warming spices, a little less salt than usual, and perhaps a peppery kick instead. In your Everyday Ayurveda experiments, you can choose to go for a curry flavor with the masala called Spring Spice Mix or for the bright taste of basil and lemon in the Spring Salts. Both deliver the tastes that balance the heavy, wet, cool qualities of springtime. Either way, you are calling on energizing herbs and spices that will support your liver in lightening its load for the coming warm weather.

SPRING SPICE MIX

Makes about ¼ cup

1 tbsp whole coriander seed
1 tsp fenugreek seed
1 tbsp whole cumin seed
1 tbsp turmeric powder
1 tbsp ginger powder
1 tsp black pepper
⅛ tsp cayenne pepper
pinch of clove powder

Dry roast the coriander, fenugreek, and cumin seeds in a heavy-bottomed pan until you can smell them, just a few minutes. Cool completely. Combine them with the rest of the spices and grind to a uniform consistency in a coffee grinder dedicated to spices or by hand with a mortar and pestle.

Using a teaspoon or funnel, transfer the spice mix to a small shaker jar with an airtight lid for storage.

SPRING SALTS

Makes ½ cup

1 tbsp finely ground pink salt
¼ cup dried lemon zest
2 tbsp dried basil
1½ tsp freshly ground black pepper
¼ tsp cayenne pepper

Mix the ingredients together in a bowl (grinding to a uniform consistency first with a mortar and pestle, if needed). Transfer to a small glass shaker jar. Some of the spring recipes will call for these seasonal salts, but you may also keep the jar on the table to use them as a condiment.

NOTE: In spring and winter, it's a good idea to keep a pepper grinder filled with pretty tricolored peppercorns on the table. You can grind up the portion for this recipe using the tabletop grinder.

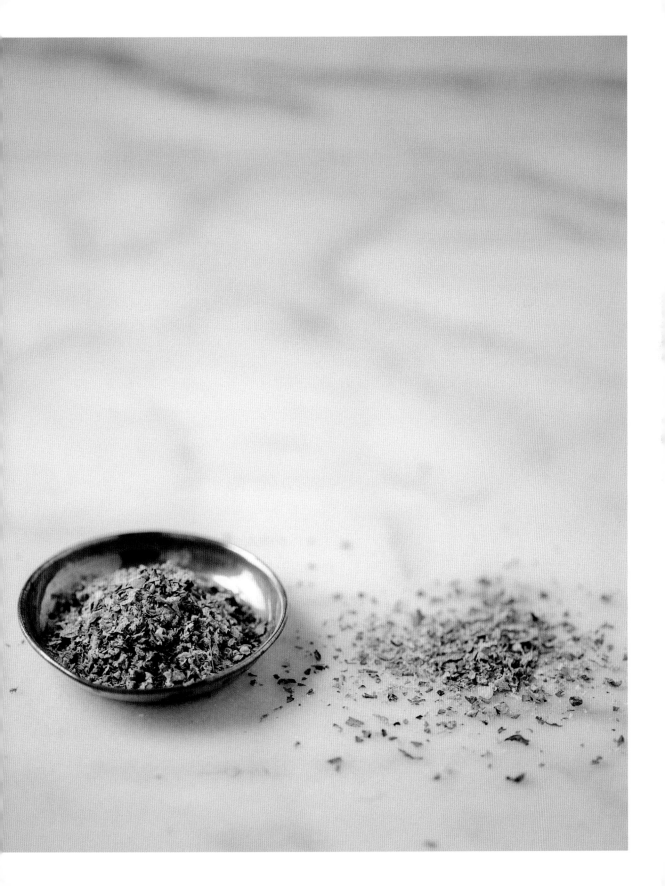

spicy black bean hummus

serves 4

Obviously, this dip is great with chips and crackers, but what about serving it with baked sweet potato wedges or parboiled carrot sticks? Or wrapped up in lettuce leaves? It pays to have some alternate dippers ready so you don't overload on the dry, rough qualities of typical snack foods.

EXTRAS

1 cup cooked black beans

2 tbsp salsa or chopped tomatoes

¼ tsp ground cumin

2 tsp fresh lemon juice

1 tsp apple cider vinegar

1 tsp olive oil

dash of salt

In a large, deep bowl, blend all the ingredients together with a hand blender until they are pureed smooth or reach your preferred texture. Serve in a decorative bowl with dippers, or a few spoonfuls on top of a Steamed Salad Bowl.

OPTIONAL FOR SERVING: Set aside 1 tsp of the salsa or chopped tomato to put on top, along with a sprig of fresh parsley.

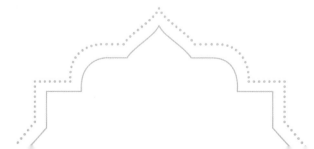

warm artichoke, spinach, and goat cheese dip

serves 2

This recipe provides the feeling of a warm, cheesy dip without the heavy, oily qualities of cow's cheese, which can be too hard to digest in spring. There are more greens than cheese here—but if you keep that quiet, no one will notice.

5 whole artichoke hearts
1 6-oz bag baby spinach
   (4 large handfuls)
½ tsp Spring Salts
1 oz goat cheese, crumbled

Preheat oven to 350 degrees. Pulse the artichoke hearts, spinach, and Spring Salts in a food processor until they reach a coarse consistency. Place the vegetables in a 16-ounce ramekin, sprinkle the goat cheese over the top, and bake for 25 minutes or until top begins to brown.

Serve with vegetable sticks, Everyday Steamed Salad Bowl, rye crackers, or rice crackers.

NOTE: If you don't own a food processor, chop the spinach and artichokes first, then use a hand blender to process them to a coarse consistency.

CHEESE IN SPRING

No matter how much you love cow's cheese, Ayurveda does not recommend it during the rainy season, especially at dinnertime, after which it will sit in your gut while you sleep. Goat's cheese lightens and warms, while cow's cheese increases heavy, dense qualities.

raisin pomegranate chutney

makes about 12 ounces

The heavy, watery nature of sweet taste must be balanced by light, dry, warming qualities in springtime. Thanks to the skin of the red grape, raisins are slightly astringent and dry, which makes them a good way to add sweetness without increasing the water element. Please note the serving size here is 1 tablespoon, just a small spoonful to accompany dinner. The intention is to counteract a dessert craving by adding a wee bit of sweet to the main meal.

1 cup raisins
½-inch piece fresh gingerroot,
    peeled and diced
½ cup pomegranate juice
juice of ½ lemon
1 tbsp raw honey
¼ tsp cardamom powder

Pulse all the ingredients in a food processor until they reach a chunky, jamlike consistency, just a few times. Transfer the chutney to a pint-size lidded container or bowl and let the flavors meld for at least 30 minutes before serving.

Store in a glass storage container in the refrigerator for up to 3 days.

THE FOOD COMBINING DANCE

Fruits mixed with other foods often do not digest well. Yet Ayurveda considers certain cooked and spiced combinations of fruits and other foods redeemable. Dried fruits that have been soaked, spiced, and cooked into a compote or chutney are easily digested, if eaten in moderation. Cardamom and ginger, as well as the process of soaking, harmonize the other ingredients in chutney. Stick to the serving size to enhance, and not disturb, your digestion.

mustard balsamic vinaigrette

serves 2–3

This dressing features a light oil to balance the heavy qualities of spring. Due to the warming actions of honey and balsamic vinegar, this dressing adds sharp and penetrating qualities to bolster the digestion and assimilation of your meal. Use a high-quality balsamic vinegar, which has less acid than cheap vinegars. Review the section on deepana and pachana (see page 40) for more ways to build the digestive fire, which may need a boost in damp weather.

2 tbsp sunflower or
   grapeseed oil
¼ cup high-quality balsamic
   vinegar
1 tsp Dijon mustard
1 tbsp raw honey dissolved
   in 1 tbsp warm water
1 tsp tamari

Shake all ingredients together in an 8-ounce jar or use a blender to whip up a double batch of this dressing.

To serve, drizzle on seasonal vegetables or on an Everyday Steamed Salad Bowl. Store in a dispenser that can be briskly shaken before serving, without leakage. Keep refrigerated.

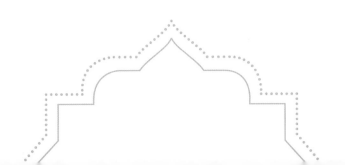

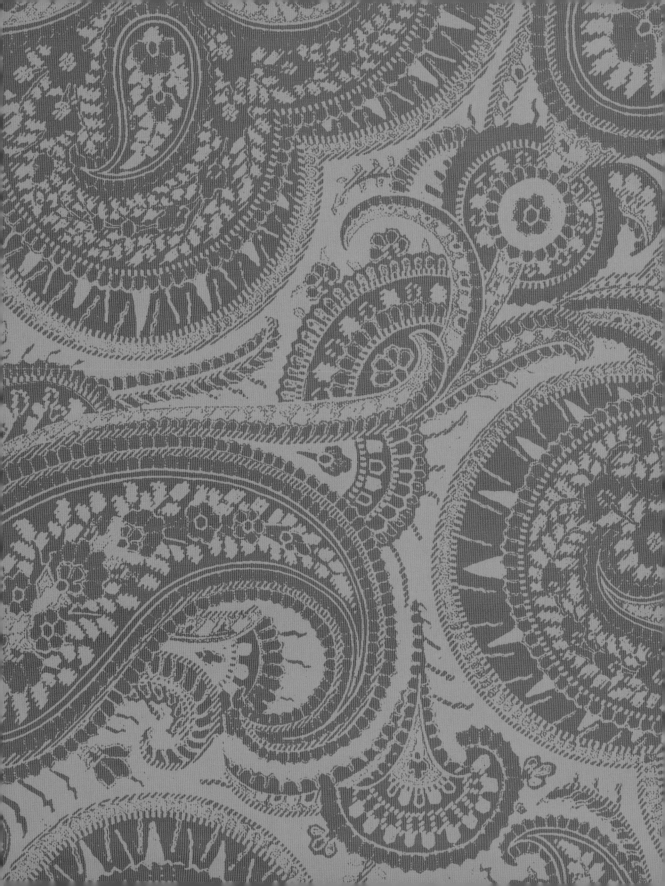

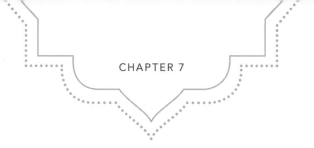

CHAPTER 7

Summer Recipes

COOLING AND CALMING FOODS TO REFRESH THE BODY ON HOT, HUMID DAYS

The garden is full, and the farmers' market is bursting with local fruits and vegetables. Your body's cravings for the heavy fats and proteins of winter and the pungency of spring naturally subside. Refreshing foods that lighten the body and keep the system cool, such as cilantro, cucumber, melon, and zucchini, will alleviate discomfort from the hot, sharp, oily qualities of heat and humidity. The summer recipes harness the bitter taste of fresh greens to cool the blood, the astringency of seasonal fruits to tone the tissues, and mildly sweet foods like fennel and coconut to balance fire in the digestive tract.

Summer Diet and Lifestyle Overview

The Elements: Fire and water
Feels Like: Hot, humid, bright

QUALITIES TO INTRODUCE/REDUCE

Introduce	*Reduce*
Cooling	Heating
Neutralizing	Sharp, acidic
Slow (relaxing)	Sharp/quick (fast-paced, intense)
Dry	Oily

POTENTIAL SIGNS AND SYMPTOMS OF IMBALANCE

Acid indigestion
Puffiness
Red skin inflammation
Irritability

TASTES TO ENJOY

Bitter
Astringent
Sweet

Summer Foods Guide

Favor foods that are cooling, calming, and slightly dry.

FOODS TO FAVOR

- Bitter and astringent vegetables, such as zucchini, broccoli, leafy greens, celery, green beans, and fennel root
- Sweet, not sour, dairy products, such as milk and ghee
- Light, neutral grains, such as quinoa, white basmati rice, and barley
- Sweet, neutral fruits, such as grapes, pomegranates, stone fruits, melons, and limes
- Cool and light proteins, such as mung beans, tofu, and (for nonvegetarians) lean white meats and fish
- Coconuts and coconut products: water, milk, meat, and sugar
- Cooling spices and herbs, such as fennel seed, coriander, cilantro, cardamom, mint, and turmeric; aloe juice

FOODS TO REDUCE

- Spicy foods
- Coffee

- Vinegar and other ferments (use balsamic vinegar in moderation)
- Alcohol (spirits and red wine are the most aggravating)
- Salty foods
- Raw tomatoes
- Raw onion
- Red meat and egg yolks
- Orange juice
- Sour dairy products, such as packaged yogurt and hard cheeses
- Heating foods, such as chilies, sour tomatoes, and honey
- Anything fried or excessively oily

SUMMER LIFESTYLE GUIDELINES
- Use coconut oil for abhyanga massage (unless your body runs cold, even in warm weather). You may add relaxing scents such as jasmine, lavender, and rose essential oils. Oil massage can be practiced morning or evening to cool down.
- Practice moderation in choosing activities and avoid overscheduling yourself.
- Engage in noncompetitive exercise, like swimming, moderate yoga, and walking.
- Take cool baths and showers.
- Stay out of the midday sun, but do enjoy time in nature. Spend time outside when the sun is lower in the sky or try moon bathing instead of sunbathing.
- Drink room temperature or cool water, not cold or ice water.

SUMMER SHOPPING LIST

VEGETABLES	FRUITS	GRAINS	FATS	SPICES
Beets	Apples	Barley	Avocados	Cardamom
Corn	Berries	Quinoa	Coconut, shredded	Coriander
Cucumbers	Dates			Fennel
Fennel	Melons	**BEANS**	Coconut milk	Turmeric
Lettuce	Peaches	Chickpeas	Coconut oil	
Summer squashes	Plums	White beans	Goat cheese	**EXTRAS**
Zucchini			Yogurt, homemade or farm-fresh	Chickpea flour
Herbs (parsley, cilantro, thyme, basil, mint, dill)				Coconut water
				Hemp protein
				Rose water

the beet queen

serves 2

Sweet and bright! This recipe produces a towering beverage; you may choose to share it or pour half into a jar to bring to work. It is great after morning exercise or to tide you over while cooking. The Beet Queen is known for clearing sluggish bowels. Use a Granny Smith apple when in season.

BREAKFAST

1 tbsp chia seeds (optional)
1 apple, cored and cut into
    quarters
½ beet, peeled and coarsely
    chopped
2–3 kale or Swiss chard leaves
    or handful of baby spinach
juice of ¼ lemon
1 cup water or coconut water
handful of parsley leaves
    (no stems)

Soak the chia seeds, if using, in a small bowl of water for 5 minutes. Using a carafe blender, put the apple chunks in the carafe first, followed by the beet, lemon juice, leafy greens (except the parsley), and optional chia seeds. Add water or coconut water. Pulse all the ingredients in the blender for 30 seconds, then process on high, adding the parsley leaves through the top as the blender is running. You may need to stop the blender and stir the solids around a few times. Blend until smooth.

The chia seeds act as a thickener, so if you want your Beet Queen to have a juicelike consistency, add more water or omit the chia seeds.

Pour into 2 glasses to serve or save half in a glass jar.

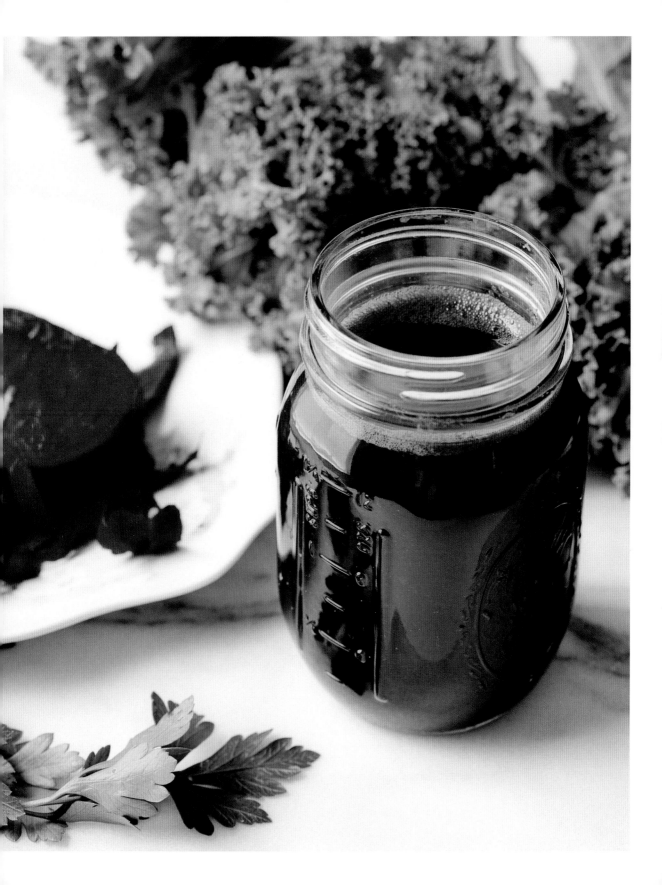

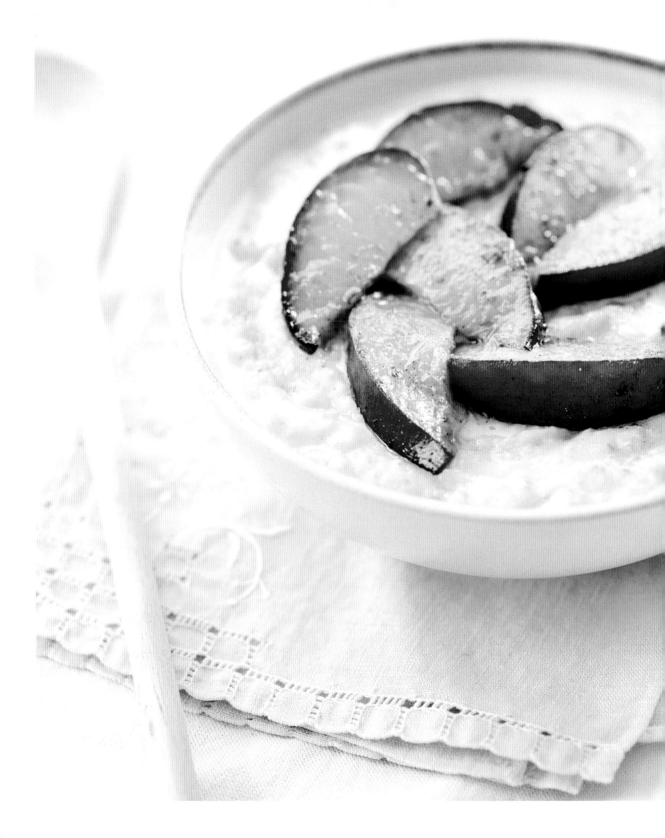

creamy coconut breakfast barley with peaches

serves 2

This meal is sweet, chewy, and satisfying—it will stick with you and nourish you all morning. Barley removes excess water from the system and is a good choice if summer humidity is making you feel puffy.

⬤⬤●⬤⬤

½ cup pearled barley

2½ cups water

1 peach, pitted and sliced

2 tsp coconut oil

1–2 pinches of cardamom

½ cup coconut milk

1 tbsp coconut sugar (optional)

Rinse the barley in a fine mesh sieve. Add it to a small pot with the water and cook, lid slightly ajar, for 25 minutes or until water is absorbed and barley is soft.

While the barley is cooking, heat the coconut oil in a small, heavy-bottomed pan over low heat. Put the peach slices in the coconut oil, sprinkle with a pinch or two of cardamom, and sauté until the edges begin to brown slightly.

Add to the cooked barley, the coconut milk, optional coconut sugar, and enough water to make it blendable with your immersion hand blender. (If you are using a carafe blender, keep the lid slightly ajar to let steam out while blending.) Process until smooth and creamy.

To serve, pour the cereal into 2 bowls and top with sautéed peaches.

RECIPES FOR PEACH SEASON

Peach season is notoriously short, so when it's at its height, make the most of it!

Peach Butter

If you have bruised or mealy peaches, substitute them for apples in the Gingered Apple Butter recipe (page 242) and waste nothing! Serve Peach Butter on top of the Creamy Coconut Breakfast Barley instead of the sautéed peach slices.

Ghee Fried Peaches with Blueberries

Follow the Ghee Fried Apples recipe (page 253), replacing the apples with peaches, and stir in a small handful of blueberries for a delicious, perfectly summery treat.

hemp protein squares

makes 6

Hemp is a balanced vegetarian source of protein, with easy-to-digest fats and a nutty flavor. Plant protein is important for those who are physically active this time of year. This no-bake recipe helps you keep your cool by delivering coconut, cardamom, and sweet taste without your having to turn on the stove. These don't do well left out in the heat, so keep them cool in the refrigerator or in an insulated lunch bag to eat sooner rather than later. Wrap them in wax paper when tucking in your bag for a snack.

BREAKFAST

¼ cup hemp protein powder

½ cup almond or sunflower butter

¼ cup unsweetened shredded coconut

1 tbsp plus 1 tsp coconut oil

¼ cup pitted Medjool dates (4–5 dates)

¼ cup dried apricots (about 6)

⅛ tsp cardamom powder

In a food processor carafe, mix together all the ingredients except 1 tsp of the coconut oil. Run the processor until the mixture forms a ball in the carafe. If it doesn't form a ball, add the remaining coconut oil and continue to process until it does. Press the mixture into a shallow 8 x 8-inch baking dish or square, lidded storage container and refrigerate until hard.

To serve, cut into 6 squares.

NOTE: Don't have a food processor? In a large mixing bowl, combine the hemp protein, cardamom, almond butter, 1 tbsp melted coconut oil, and 1 tbsp maple syrup together with a fork until well blended. Refrigerate as above.

HEMP PROTEIN

Hemp protein is simply ground hemp seed, which retains its fiber and omega fats. Unlike some protein powders, in which a whole food has been separated into different parts, hemp protein remains a whole food. The body is more likely to recognize, metabolize, and assimilate a whole food than one that has been separated.

SEASONAL RECIPES AND ROUTINES

lemon rice picnic with beetroot palya and cucumber raita

Each of these recipes can stand on its own, but should you have occasion to provide a special picnic for friends and family, the three dishes make up a classic south Indian meal. I have learned how to cook these dishes by observing householders who were kind enough to teach me and Ayurvedic cooks as well, to note the differences between everyday cooking and medicinal cooking. Here I fuse the two: I have changed the recipes slightly, in line with Ayurvedic sensitivities, but the dishes are still quite authentic and bring the tastes of Ayurveda's roots to your kitchen. It gives me happiness to share this feast with you.

LEMON RICE

serves 2

When you don't want to heat up your kitchen on a hot summer day, mix up this rice meal using leftover rice and just a few minutes of stove-top cooking time.

1 cup raw basmati rice

1 tbsp coconut oil

½ tsp mustard seeds

1 tbsp peanuts

2 tbsp cashews

¼ tsp hing (asafetida)

½ tsp turmeric powder

½-inch piece fresh gingerroot, grated

2–3 red chilies, dried

juice of 1 small or ½ large lemon

1 handful cilantro leaves, roughly chopped

sea salt to taste

In a large saucepan, combine the basmati rice with 2 cups boiling water and cook at low heat, covered, for 10–15 minutes or until water is absorbed. Allow to cool, so the grains stay separate. Leftover rice works well also.

Heat oil over medium heat in a heavy-bottomed skillet. Add mustard seeds until they begin to splutter and pop, then add peanuts, cashews, hing, turmeric powder, grated ginger, and chilies. Sauté for a few minutes, just until peanuts and cashews begin to brown. Remove from heat.

Put the cooled rice into a large serving bowl. Add lemon juice, cilantro, spiced nut mixture, and salt to the rice and mix slowly with your hands so as not to break the rice grains.

Serve at room temperature, alongside Beetroot Palya and a dollop of Cucumber Mint Raita, or pack it in your tiffin (the Indian stainless steel container with a latching top) for a picnic lunch.

BEETROOT PALYA

serves 2

Palya is the Kannada word used in the state of Maharashtra for vegetables fried with spices, though every region in south India has its own name for this dish. This versatile recipe often features shredded or diced cabbage, carrots, green beans, or okra. Frequently it also includes onion and urad dal, but this Ayurvedic version omits those foods and uses only the traditional mustard seed and shredded coconut. Once you get the hang of this recipe, start experimenting with any vegetable you have on hand. The amount of water will vary by vegetable, so start with less than the ½ cup in this recipe and add a few ounces more during cooking, as needed.

1   tbsp coconut oil

1   tsp mustard seeds

pinch asafetida (hing) powder
    (optional)

2   cups peeled, finely diced
    beets

½ cup shredded coconut

¼ tsp cinnamon

1   tsp. salt

½ cup water

Warm the coconut oil in a large frying pan over medium heat. Add the mustard seeds and asafetida powder, if using, and fry in the oil for 2-3 minutes. Cover the pan with a lid so the seeds don't escape when they pop. Add the diced beets and shredded coconut and fry for a few seconds more, stirring to distribute the oil and spices throughout. Add the cinnamon and salt, then the water. Stir, cover, turn the heat down to low, and simmer for 10 minutes.

Serve alongside Lemon Rice.

CUCUMBER MINT RAITA

serves 4

Often the raita found in Indian restaurants contains raw onion, a pungent food to be moderated in summer. This version is gentler on the system and acts as a digestive aid. Should you desire more exciting flavors, a few spice variations are listed. It's best made fresh so the cucumber is crisp.

1   large or 2 small cucumbers

¼ tsp salt

¼ tsp pepper

1   cup organic whole milk
    yogurt

¼ tsp coriander, fennel, or cumin
    powder (optional)

mint sprigs for garnish (optional)

Peel the cucumber with a vegetable peeler, leaving a few strips of skin for color. Cut it in half lengthwise. Scrape out and discard the seeds. Grate the cucumber halves with a large box grater. In a medium-sized bowl, mix the grated cucumber, ground spice if using, salt, and pepper into the yogurt until well blended. Garnish with sprigs of mint on top, if you like.

Serve raita beside grains and vegetables or pack it in its own container for the Lemon Rice Picnic.

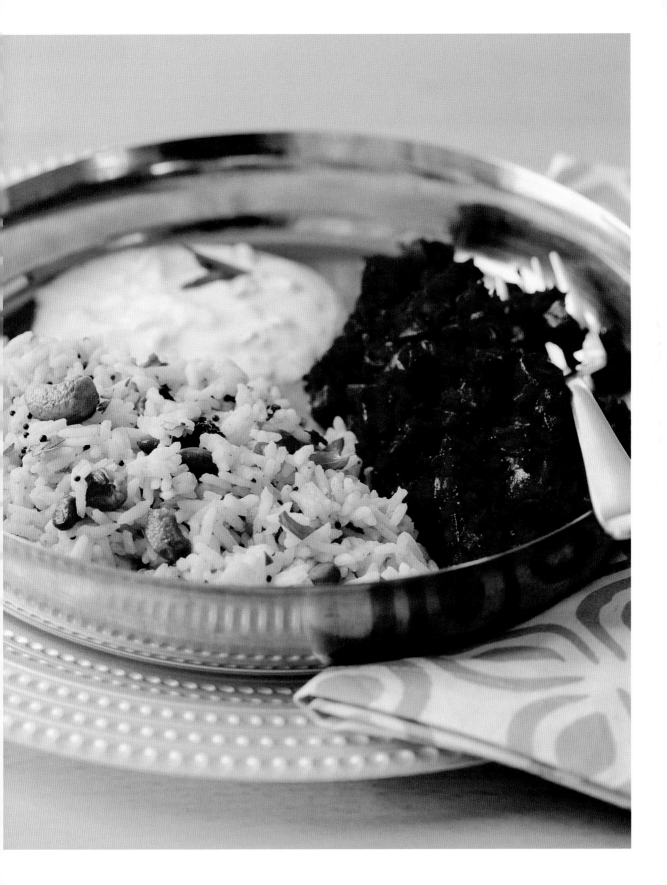

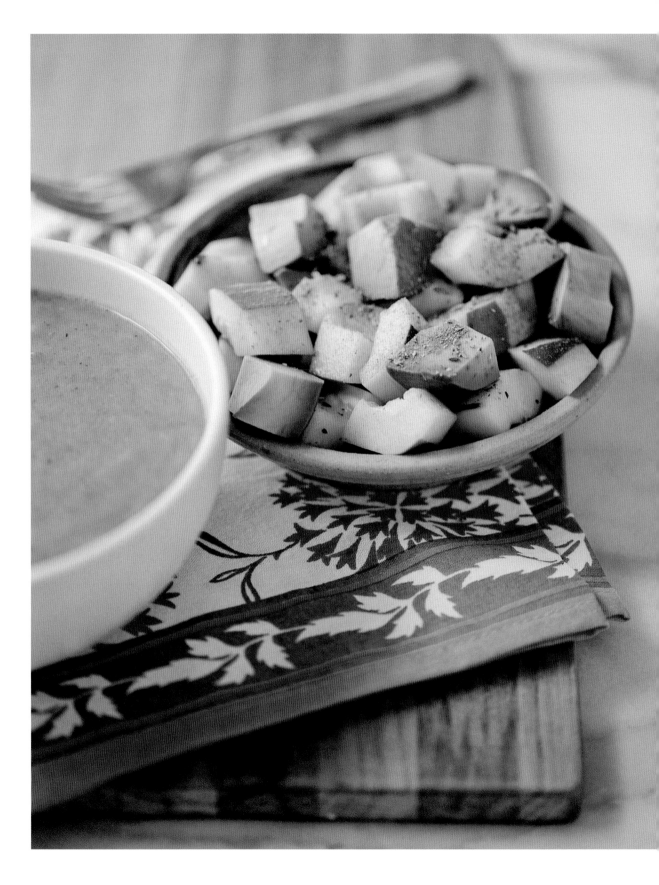

only zucchini soup with avocado and cucumber salad

serves 2

Only Zucchini Soup will amaze you with its creaminess. Zucchini has astringent and bitter qualities, which benefit the body greatly in summer. This soup-and-salad combo comes together quickly and offers you lots of fresh vegetables.

ONLY ZUCCHINI SOUP

2 medium zucchini or summer squash

1 tsp ghee

1 cup water

¼ tsp salt

Cut the zucchini or yellow squash in half lengthwise, then into ½-inch-thick half moons. In a medium-size saucepan, fry the zucchini or squash in the ghee over medium heat until tender, 5–7 minutes. Add water and salt. Cook on medium heat until warm. Remove from heat. With an immersion hand blender, process until smooth.

AVOCADO AND CUCUMBER SALAD

1 medium cucumber

1 avocado

½ tsp Summer Spice Mix (see page 203)

pinch of salt

¼ lime

Peel the cucumber, leaving a few long stripes of skin on for texture and color. Cut in half lengthwise, scrape out the seeds with a teaspoon, and chop the flesh into cubes.

Halve the avocado lengthwise and twist to separate the halves. Refrigerate the half with the seed still in it in an airtight container. Cut the other half into cubes and scoop them out of the peel with a large spoon.

In a small bowl, combine the cucumber and avocado cubes. Sprinkle with spice mix and salt, squeeze the lime over them, and mix all together.

Serve immediately alongside Only Zucchini Soup.

ayur-corn chowder with easy chana dosa

serves 2

Unlike its namesake, usually made with milk and flour, this chowder is sweet and light to balance the oily feeling of humid weather. Round out your meal with Easy Chana Dosa for dipping. Omit the red pepper if you are prone to a hot internal environment.

●●●●●

AYUR-CORN CHOWDER

2–3 ears corn

½ cup yellow summer squash

2 cups unsweetened rice milk

1 tsp ghee

½ tsp Summer Spice Mix (see page 203)

2 tsp finely diced red bell pepper (optional)

salt and pepper to taste

chopped cilantro for garnish

In a steaming basket in a large covered pot, steam 2–3 ears of corn for 10 minutes. Remove the ears from the heat, cool a bit, then remove the kernels by sliding a knife down the sides of the ears. You'll get about 1 cup, depending on the size of the ears.

Use the large pot to boil the summer squash in the rice milk for 10 minutes.

Add the ghee, ½ cup of the corn, and the spice mix to the squash and rice milk in the saucepan. With an immersion hand blender, process until smooth. Now stir in the remaining ½ cup corn and the diced bell pepper, if using, and heat for 10 minutes more.

Add salt and pepper to taste and serve in 2 bowls, garnishing with chopped cilantro.

EASY CHANA DOSA

makes 4–5

Chana means "chickpea," and this recipe calls for chickpea (or garbanzo bean) flour, a very dense and gluten-free flour that results from simply grinding the whole bean. In a damp or humid season, chickpea flour is balancing for its dry quality and easy to use. These dosas pack a lot of protein, and you may find that just one dosa will do at a meal. They also pair well with Cilantro Mint Chutney (see page 202) at any meal, even breakfast. To keep it really simple, omit the grated zucchini—and they will cook faster.

½ tsp salt

1 cup chickpea flour

¾ cup water

1 cup grated zucchini

4–5 tbsp chopped fresh cilantro

ghee for cooking

In a small mixing bowl, mix the salt with the flour. Slowly blend the water into the flour until the mixture has the consistency of pancake batter. Stir in the grated zucchini.

Warm a large ceramic nonstick skillet over medium-high heat. Flick a few drops of water on the pan—when it sizzles the pan is ready. Pour ⅓ cup of the dosa batter into the pan,

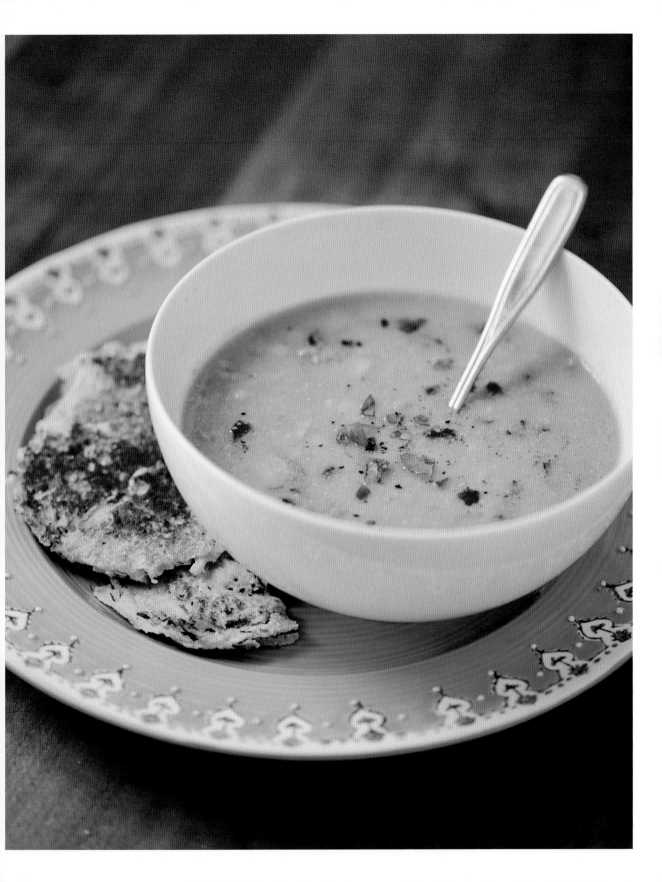

slightly tilt the pan, and spread the batter in circles with the back of a large spoon until the dosa is thin, about 7 inches round. Sprinkle 1 tbsp of fresh cilantro evenly over the batter. When it begins to look dry on top, drizzle ½ tsp of ghee over the dosa, then check to see that the bottom is browning. Flip it a few times and cook until both sides are brown. Each dosa takes about 5 minutes to cook.

NOTE: This frying technique is much like the one in the Everyday Dosa recipe, but it will still require a bit of practice. A ceramic nonstick pan makes this dish easier to execute, but you may botch the first dosa before you get the heat right. Once you are familiar with the temperament of your pan and your burner, your dosa technique will gel.

maha quinoa salad

serves 3-4

You might happily eat this salad all the time as your main summer meal—hence the word *maha* in the name, meaning "great." Quinoa is high in plant protein and is on the light and dry side. If you have fresh herbs, these can be stirred in at the end before serving. Parsley and cilantro are my favorites in the Maha Quinoa Salad.

FOR THE QUINOA

- 2 cups water
- 1 cup white quinoa (or white with a little red mixed in for color)
- 2 cups mixed summer vegetables (zucchini, carrots, bok choy, green beans, and/or sugar snap peas), coarsely chopped
- chopped fresh parsley for garnish

FOR THE DRESSING

- 1 large or 2 small lemons
- 3 tbsp olive or hemp oil
- 1 tsp salt
- 1 tsp Summer Spice Mix (see page 203)

MAKE THE QUINOA:

In a medium saucepan, bring 2 cups of water to a boil. Add quinoa and simmer covered on low heat for 10 minutes. Add chopped vegetables on top of the cooking quinoa, cover to steam, and cook 10 minutes more. Remove the pan from the heat, fluff the quinoa and vegetables together with a fork, and leave uncovered until cool.

MAKE THE DRESSING:

Juice the lemons into a small mixing bowl. Whisk in the olive or hemp oil, salt, and spice mix until well blended or shake together in an 8-ounce jar.

Pour the dressing over the quinoa when fully cooled and mix together with a fork.

Serve as a stand-alone entrée, garnished with chopped fresh parsley, or with a side of Herbed Hummus (page 200).

VARIATION: QUINOA TABOULI

Cook the quinoa as in the recipe, omit the mixed vegetables and spice mix, stir in ½–1 cup of chopped fresh parsley and 6 halved cherry tomatoes after the quinoa cools, and you've got Quinoa Tabouli.

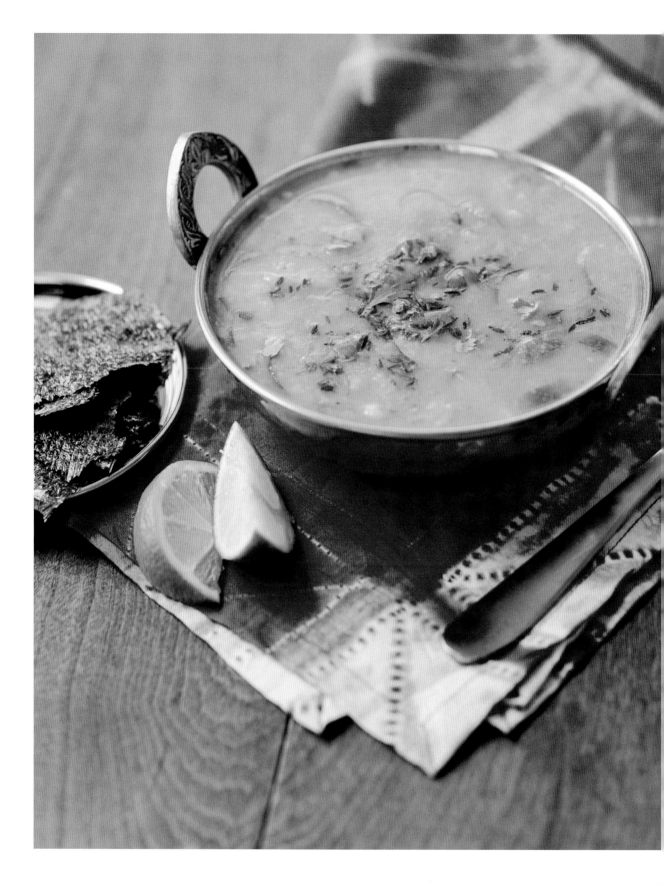

detox dal soup

serves 4-6

This dal is thinner and lighter than the cool-weather version, Warming Tomato Dal, on page 255; it contains cooling spices, summer vegetables, and a good hit of lime for a refreshing, satisfying meal. It will cook up quickly to minimize stove-top time on a hot day. Detox Dal Soup helps the body get rid of ama, unwanted toxins. To enjoy it in other seasons, simply swap out the seasonal spice mix and add a seasonally appropriate vegetable.

1 cup yellow split mung beans

6 cups water

1 tsp turmeric powder

1 tsp coriander powder

1 tsp Summer Spice Mix (see page 203)

2 small zucchini

½ tsp salt (optional)

2 tsp coconut oil

1 tsp cumin seeds

small handful fresh curry leaf

juice of ½ lime

2 tbsp chopped cilantro for garnish (optional)

In a large saucepan, heat 4 cups of the water over high heat until it boils. While the water is heating, rinse the split mung beans in cool water until the water runs clear. Add the mung beans, turmeric powder, coriander powder, and spice mix to the saucepan. Turn heat down to low, cover with the lid slightly ajar, and simmer for 20 minutes.

Cut the zucchini lengthwise, then into half moons. Add the zucchini to the pot and bring the water to a boil again. Add the remaining 2 cups of water and salt, partially cover again. No need to stir. Simmer for another 10 minutes.

In a small frying pan, heat the coconut oil over medium heat, add cumin seeds and curry leaf, and sauté until you can smell the spices, just 2-3 minutes. Add the tempered spices to the dal for the last 5 minutes of the cooking time. Remove from heat and stir in the lime juice.

Serve in bowls with a topping of the fresh cilantro or with a lime wedge, perhaps a side of Toasted Nori (page 265).

NOTE: If your dal is not as creamy as you would like, soften the beans by blending the hot dal with an immersion hand blender or an old-fashioned eggbeater for just 5-10 seconds before you add the vegetables.

CURRY LEAF

Curry leaf is a staple in many south Indian dishes. Curry leaf is known to support the liver, balance blood sugar, and help the digestive system clean out unwanted particles. Indian groceries often have fresh curry leaf, and you can freeze the leaves if you buy more than you can use immediately. If you live in a warm climate, I recommend growing curry leaf yourself.

steamed zucchini noodles
with yogurt dill sauce

serves 2

Zucchini noodles are fun to make and quick when you use a julienne peeler, found at many kitchen stores. This recipe gives you a great way to eat up those abundant zucchinis from the summer garden and to benefit from their cooling nature. Sub in a julienned carrot or yellow squash for beauty. The noodles also go great with Whipped Tahini Sauce, accompanied by Cilantro Mint Chutney or in a Noodle Bowl (see pages 217, 202, 264).

SUPPER

FOR THE NOODLES

1 cup water

2 small or medium-size
   zucchini

FOR THE SAUCE

¼ cup chopped fresh dill

1 cup organic whole milk
   yogurt

1 tbsp fresh lemon juice

½ tsp turmeric powder

½ tsp salt

freshly ground pepper to taste

MAKE THE NOODLES:

Pour water into a medium saucepan with steamer basket. Bring to a boil.

Draw the julienne peeler down the zucchinis lengthwise to form noodles. Pile the noodles into the steamer basket, cover, and steam for 3-4 minutes. The noodles should be al dente. Drain into a colander immediately.

MAKE THE SAUCE:

In a small mixing bowl, whisk all the ingredients together with a fork until well blended.

To serve, divide the warm noodles into 2 bowls and pour the yogurt sauce over each serving.

FINDING FRESH YOGURT

It is important to buy fresh yogurt when it is available—farmers' markets often have locally made yogurt for sale—or learn to make your own at home. The longer yogurt sits, the more it ferments, making the yogurt sour. Sour taste is sharp in quality and heating for the body, which is not what we are going for in the summer. Packaged yogurt is never as balancing for the system as fresh, whole milk yogurt, which is more sweet in taste.

SEASONAL RECIPES AND ROUTINES

fresh fennel and dill soup

serves 2

Fennel has the cooling, soothing properties to balance the sometimes intense qualities of summer weather. Whip up this simple vegetable soup for an easy supper that will help you relax.

1   fennel bulb

1   tsp ghee

2   large kale or Swiss chard
    leaves

3   cups water

1   tsp salt

½   cup cooked white or
    garbanzo beans or raw
    mung bean sprouts

1   tbsp finely chopped fresh
    dill (or dried)

Chop the fennel bulb into thin slices, as you would an onion. In a medium saucepan sauté the slices in ghee for about 5 minutes. Cut the kale or chard leaves into thin strips and stir in. Add the water, salt, and beans. (If you are using dried dill, add it in as well.) Simmer for 20 minutes covered. Remove from heat and stir in the fresh dill.

Serve this soup by itself for a simple supper or with an Easy Chana Dosa on the side if you are very hungry.

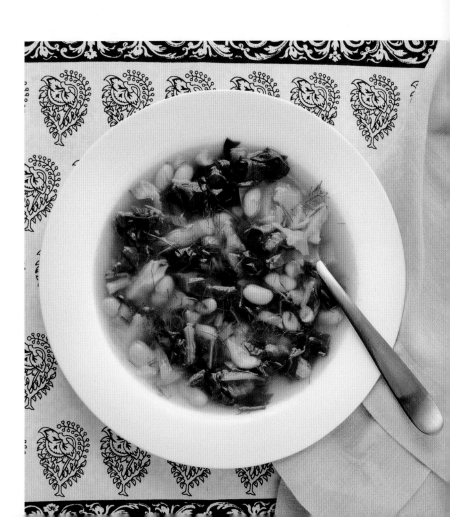

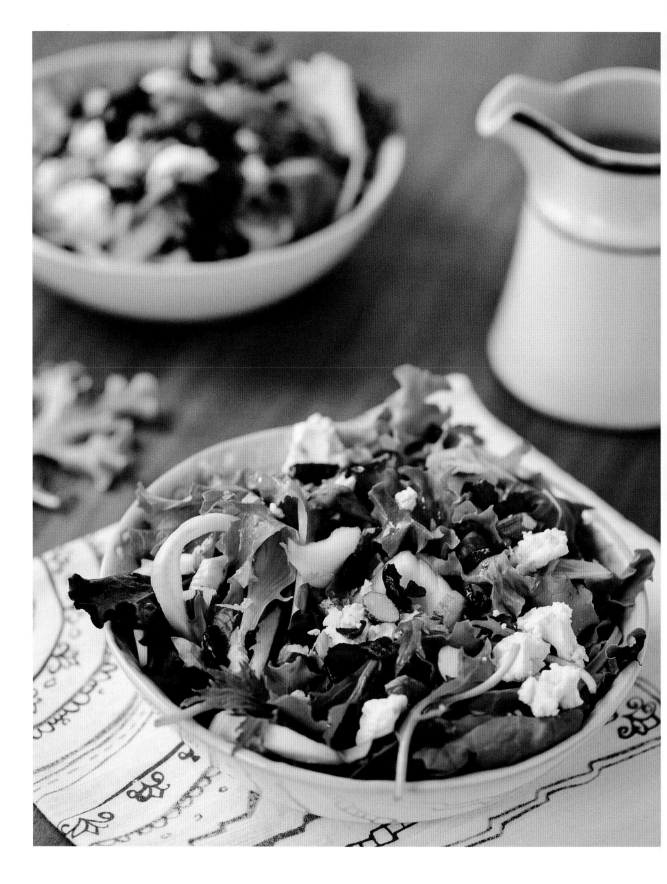

kate's only salad

serves 2

I don't often eat raw, cold salad anymore. As I learned that my body digested warm, cooked food better, salad no longer appealed to me. In the heat of summer, however, this shaved fennel salad with chèvre remains a favorite; it's colorful, cool, and sweet. All of these characteristics balance the irritability that hot weather may cause in the body. The astringent, bitter qualities of cranberries balance humidity by reducing the water in your system, while fennel balances heat with the cooling effect of its sweet licorice taste.

SUPPER

1 fennel bulb

1 head romaine or red leaf lettuce, chopped, or ½ lb mesclun greens

2 tbsp olive, sunflower, or grapeseed oil

2 tbsp fine balsamic vinegar

¼ cup chèvre

¼ cup chopped almonds or toasted sunflower seeds

¼ cup dried cranberries

Cut the woody tops off the fennel bulb (you can save them for flavoring soups or broth). Cut the fennel bulb into thin slivers with a sharp knife. In a large salad bowl, toss the slivered fennel with the greens. Divide into two wide bowls. Drizzle 1 tbsp oil and 1 tbsp vinegar over each bowl of greens. With a fork, crumble 2 tbsp of the chèvre into each bowl. If it is too soft to crumble, put the chèvre in the freezer for a few minutes.

To serve, sprinkle the almonds or sunflower seeds and cranberries on top of each salad.

OPTIONAL SERVING NOTES: Top with grated beet for added color. When beet greens are available, I steam them and enjoy them with chèvre, almonds, and cranberries.

BALSAMIC VINEGAR

You'll know low-quality balsamic vinegar because it comes in a big jug and costs a lot less than high-quality balsamic—but it also has a higher acid content, which is not advised for most in the hot months. Fine balsamic vinegar has been reduced, a slow cooking process—like caramelizing onions—that turns acidity to sweetness. Fine balsamic will offer a sweet taste, only slightly sour, with qualities more soothing than the sharp ones of an acidic vinegar.

fruit salad trio

serves 1

Most travelers to India, where fruits can be easier to come by than vegetables, will enjoy a fruit salad at breakfast time. This treat makes a light breakfast in warm weather, when the appetite is small, and also stands in for supper in hot weather. It is best to combine fruits that have similar qualities, such as mixed citrus (heating and sour for brightening winter doldrums), mixed berries (astringent and cleansing when they are in season), or mixed sweet fruits (cooling in late summer and early fall).

Enjoy each of these salads on their own, in season, for maximum benefit. Except for the combination of dates and milk, most raw fruits can create a sour effect in the stomach when mixed with other foods, so it is best to eat fruit salad alone.

NOTE: Mixed fruits at night is an Ayurvedic home remedy for sluggish bowels. If you have this problem, try a fruit salad for dinner to get things moving tomorrow.

TREATS

SEASONAL RECIPES AND ROUTINES

CITRUS SALAD

- 1 orange, sectioned and chopped
- ½ grapefruit, sectioned and chopped
- 2 dried pineapple rings, diced
- 2 tbsp coconut water
- 1 squeeze fresh lime juice on top

BERRY SALAD

- ½ cup blueberries
- ½ cup raspberries
- ½ cup chopped strawberries
- 1 tbsp dried cranberries
- 2 tbsp pomegranate juice

SWEET SALAD

- ½ chopped cored apple
- 1 chopped cored pear
- ½ cup halved red grapes
- 2 dates, pitted and diced
- 2 tbsp apple juice
- mint leaves for garnish

In a small bowl, toss the fruits together with the liquid and let stand for 20-30 minutes.

Serve by itself as a meal.

THE BANANA STANDS ALONE

Ripe banana is dense and moist. Notice there is no banana in these salads, or mixed into any recipe, for that matter. Bananas digest best when enjoyed on their own and you'll find are quite satisfying this way.

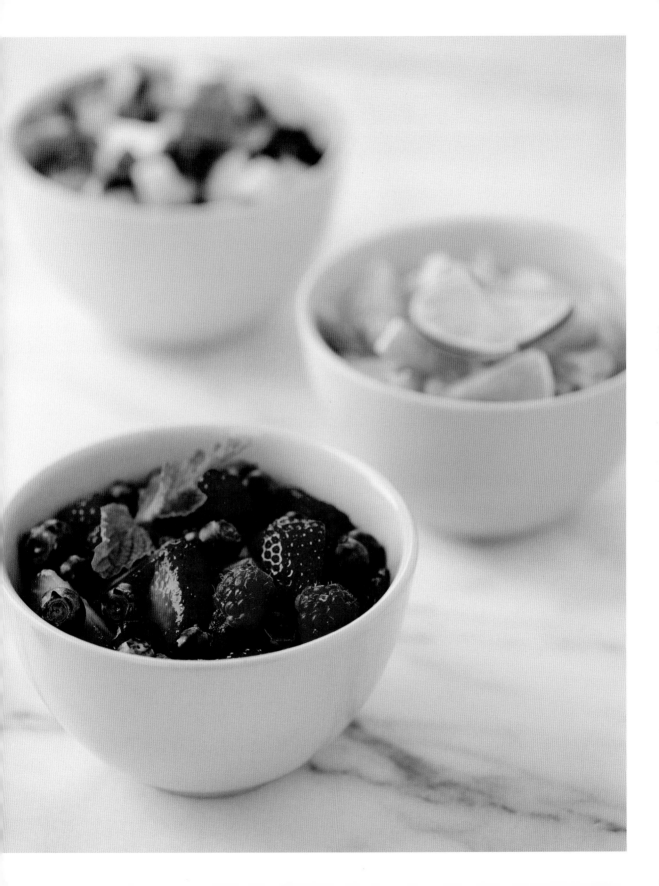

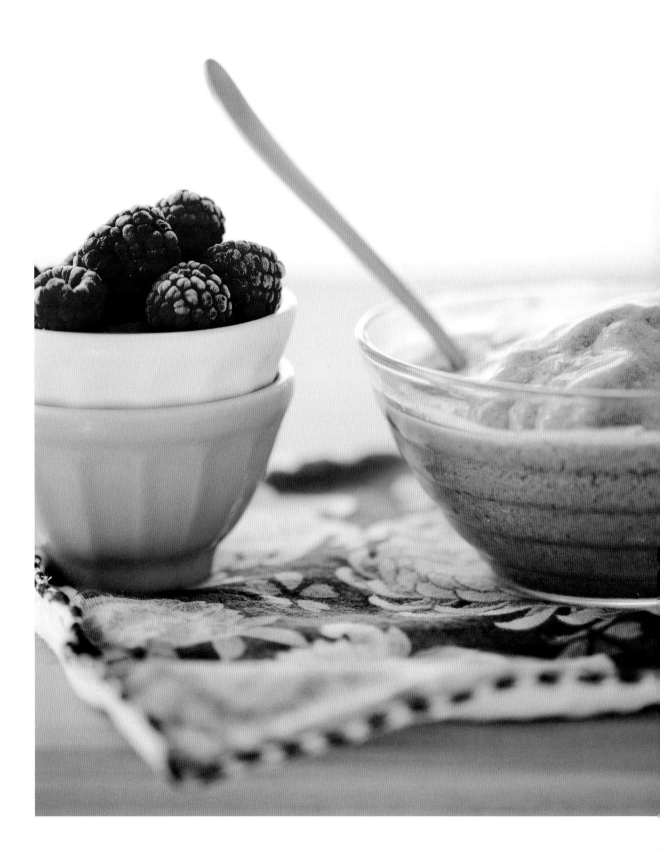

ananda-coco

serves 2

Meet your new favorite summer frozen treat: Ananda-Coco, or coconut milk ice cream. While icy foods of any sort are not recommended in Ayurveda, this recipe balances the cold by integrating ginger and is better for you than most frozen treats. It is best to have this one only on occasion as a special indulgence, when the weather is very hot. *Ananda* means "bliss" in Sanskrit, and although yoga philosophy tells us bliss does not result from an object, such as frozen treats, you might be fooled. But be forewarned: eating Ananda-Coco too often will result in a cold belly, not long-term bliss. Make your own and make it to order, as it won't freeze as well as ice cream.

1 cup canned coconut milk

½-inch piece fresh gingerroot, peeled and roughly chopped, or ½ tsp ginger powder

1 cup frozen berries (strawberries, raspberries, blueberries, etc.)

2 tbsp maple syrup or coconut sugar

1 tsp pure vanilla extract

2–3 ice cubes to thicken texture (optional)

In a blender, pulse together the coconut milk and ginger until finely mixed. Add the berries, maple syrup or coconut sugar, and vanilla extract to the blender carafe and pulse just until smooth. With the blender running, add the ice, cube by cube, if desired, until the mixture reaches a texture similar to that of sorbet or soft ice cream.

Over time, see if you can adjust to eating a less "frozen" frozen treat, reducing the number of ice cubes you use so your stomach can break it down more easily. It takes a little getting used to, but eventually you'll find that fully frozen is not as appealing as comfortably cool.

FREEZE YOUR OWN BERRIES

Fresh food is far superior to frozen. But if you live in berry country, you know how short the season is and are probably in the habit of picking and freezing your own organic berries. The care and attention you give to preserving some of your bumper crop can extend the season another month, and it also infuses prana into your fruits, but it is better not to eat foods that have been frozen much longer than that.

coconut rice pudding

serves 2

Rice pudding, known as *kheer*, often appears on holy festival days when gods and goddesses are being honored in temples and in celebratory households. Servings of this rich sweet are offered to the deities and to the pilgrims in small dishes, as part of a feast served on a banana leaf, or doled out of buckets and clay urns right into people's hands. The Ayurvedic version is much lighter than the holiday fare and can be consumed more often as a nourishing dessert. Coconut Rice Pudding can be served warm as well as cool, depending on the weather.

1 cup cooked white jasmine rice

1 cup coconut milk

2 dates, pitted and chopped

2 tsp coconut sugar or maple syrup

10 almonds, soaked and chopped or ground

¼ tsp cardamom powder

fresh mint leaves to garnish

In a medium saucepan heat the rice and coconut milk together over medium-high heat until boiling. Stir in the chopped dates, coconut sugar or maple syrup, almonds, and cardamom powder. Simmer, covered, on low heat for 15 minutes.

To serve, ladle into your guest's open hand. Or, divide into 2 decorative bowls and garnish with fresh mint.

cardamom limeade

serves 2

Together cardamom and lime juice make an exceptionally cool and refreshing drink. This beverage promises to calm irritable, overheated moods.

3 cups water

¼ cup lime juice (juice of 2–3 limes)

¼ tsp cardamom powder

1 tbsp coconut sugar dissolved in 1 tbsp hot water

Mix together all of the ingredients in a small pitcher or 32-ounce glass jar.

Serve in 2 tall glasses with 2 ice cubes per glass.

A BALANCING BEVERAGE SAVES THE DAY

Rachel came to see me when she was experiencing low energy levels and having trouble making it through a workday without eating junk food. She was accustomed to having coffee and a cookie when that three o'clock low point came around. She enjoyed the chance to get up from her desk for a few minutes, go get coffee, and come back with a treat for the last few hours of work. We talked about managing highs and lows by eating regular meals, not at the desk, and after a few months, Rachel was stopping work midday to eat a nice lunch and making it to dinner without an afternoon cookie. When she started having uncomfortable acid stomach symptoms during or after dinner, we noticed it was on the days when she still had coffee. I suggested she try drinking Cardamon Limeade instead of coffee when she craved an afternoon pick-me-up. Rachel got in the habit of making a Cardamom Limeade in the morning and bringing this neutralizing, cooling beverage in a jar from home. She no longer experiences acid stomach discomfort at dinnertime.

cukamint mocktail

makes 2 tall ones or 4 tumblers

Alcohol increases the sharp, hot, penetrating qualities we already experience in summer, arguably more than any other food, so here's a cool cocktail to quench your thirst without the booze. Getting in the swing of new habits is easier when you have something delicious to enjoy. This drink looks nice in a tumbler; put in just enough ice—two cubes per glass—to make a tinkling sound when you serve them but not enough to freeze the drinkers' bellies.

2 cucumbers, peeled, sliced lengthwise, and deseeded

a few sprigs fresh mint

2 cups coconut water

juice of 1 lime

lime wedges for garnish

In a blender carafe, blend cucumbers and mint sprigs with 1 cup of the coconut water for 1 minute, until liquefied. Then add the remaining coconut water and the lime juice to the carafe and blend again to combine.

Serve cool, pouring into 2 tall glasses or 4 tumblers, over 2 ice cubes per glass, garnishing each with a lime wedge.

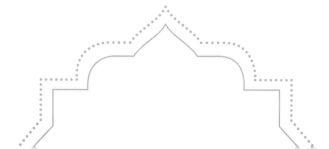

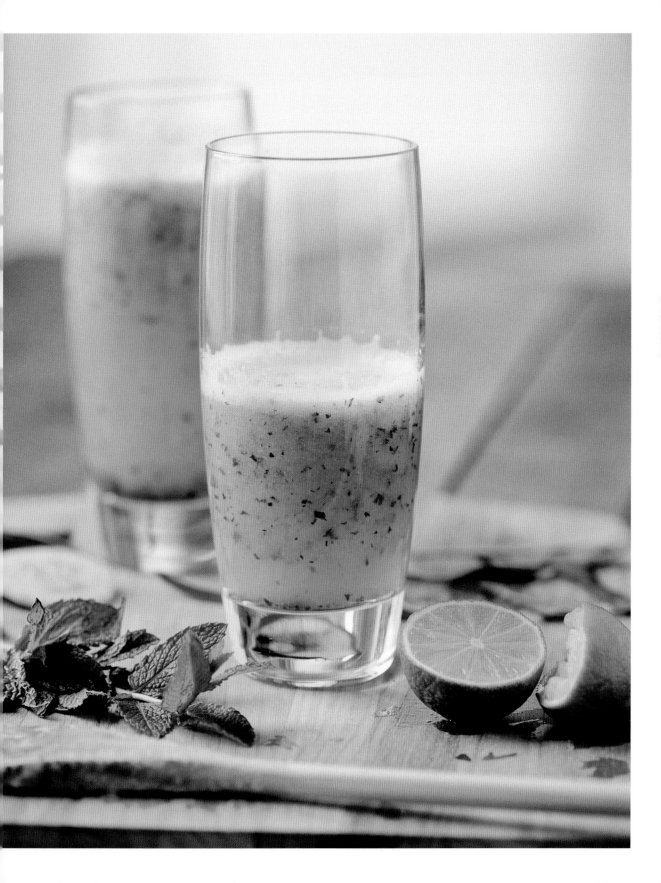

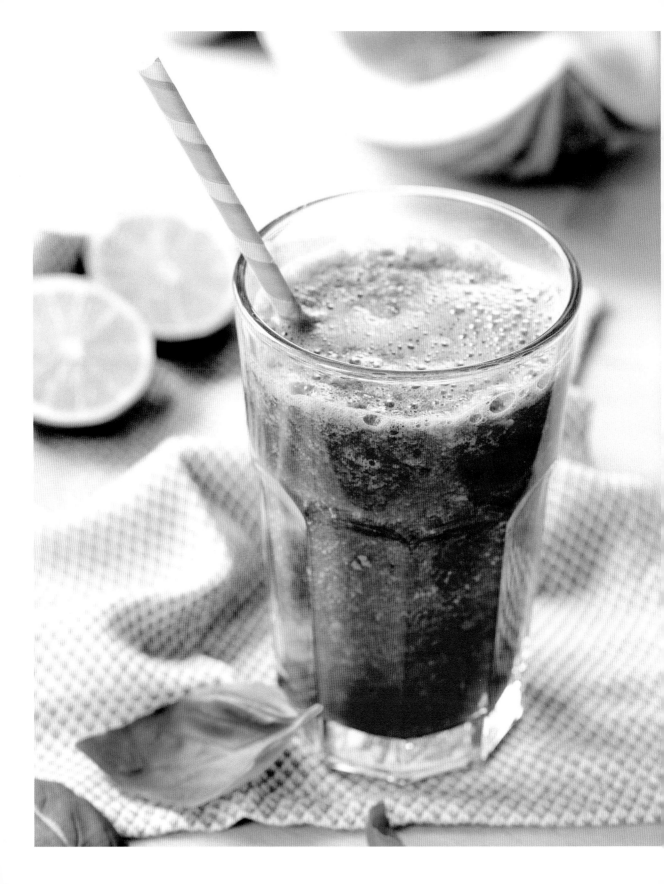

basil melon cooler

serves 4

Melon is delicious, hydrating, and cooling. However, melon does not digest well with other foods, so it's best to drink Basil Melon Cooler at least an hour before a meal. It's great as a predinner pick-me-up. Try substituting mint leaves for the basil.

4 cups chopped, deseeded
   watermelon, honeydew
   melon, or cantaloupe
4 large basil leaves
¼ tsp ginger powder
juice of 1 lime
¼–½ cup water
3–4 ice cubes (optional)
basil leaves and lime
   wedges for garnish

Put the chopped melon, 4 basil leaves, ginger powder, and lime juice in a blender carafe along with ¼ cup of the water. Blend on high speed until the basil has become green flecks. For a smoothie texture, add the ice cubes; if you prefer it more liquid, omit the ice and add up to ¼ cup more of water. Blend again until smooth.

Serve in 4 glasses, each garnished with 1 fresh basil leaf and 1 lime wedge.

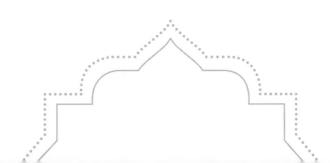

herbed hummus

makes 32 ounces (2 batches)

Store-bought hummus contains a lot of canola oil. If you take the time to make a batch yourself, yours will be chock-full of whole foods instead: pure olive oil and tahini, plus any fresh and vital herbs you'd like for flavoring. If you don't digest fats well, you can reduce the tahini and olive oil by half and add ¼ cup of the chickpea cooking water to thin the hummus out. This is a batch-sized recipe; it's great for entertaining and potlucks, served with vegetable spears, rye crackers, and rice crackers.

2 cups dried chickpeas

8 cups water

¼ cup olive oil

¼ cup fresh lemon juice (juice of 1–2 lemons)

¼ cup tahini

2 tsp sea salt, or to taste

½ cup fresh herbs, roughly chopped (cilantro, parsley, basil, rosemary, etc.)

Soak the dried chickpeas overnight. Rinse the chickpeas and simmer in a large pot with 8 cups fresh water for about 2 hours. (You can leave them unattended.) When the skins start to come off and you can squish the chickpeas between your fingers, they are ready. Put the chickpeas in a food processor or blender carafe, reserving any excess cooking water. Add the olive oil, lemon juice, tahini, and sea salt. If needed, add a few tablespoons of the reserved cooking water to process the chickpeas, enough to blend them to a smooth consistency. Add the fresh herbs and pulse until combined. (If you're using a quart-sized carafe, you may have to process the hummus in 2 batches and mix them together at the end.)

Serve in a wide bowl drizzled with olive oil, or refrigerate in storage containers for up to 5 days.

NOTE: Have you ever tried warm hummus? It's delicious. Warm the hummus in a pan on the stovetop and serve with rye or rice crackers, on an Everyday Steamed Salad Bowl, in a wrap, or with cucumber spears.

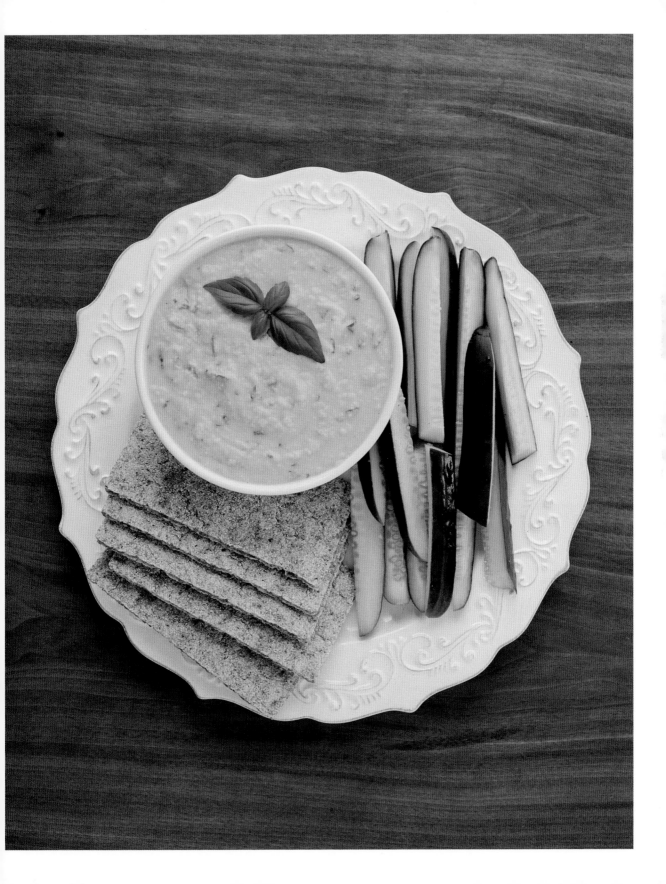

cilantro mint chutney

makes about 2 cups

This chutney brings a fresh, cool taste experience to any meal. It goes well with dals, kichari, rice dishes, and vegetables. The recipe keeps it simple—it's just herbs and coconut, really—so it combines well with most meals. In summer, serving a hearty spoonful on the side is always recommended.

½ cup fresh lemon juice

¼ cup purified water

1 bunch fresh cilantro

1 bunch fresh mint

½ cup unsweetened dried coconut

¼ cup fresh gingerroot, peeled and coarsely chopped

2 tsp raw honey (optional)

1 tsp sea salt

½ tsp freshly ground black pepper

In a food processor or carafe blender, process the lemon juice, water, cilantro, and mint until the cilantro is coarsely chopped. Add the rest of the ingredients and blend until smooth.

Store covered in the refrigerator for up to 1 week.

NOTE: You can also make pure mint or pure cilantro chutney and enjoy the flavors separately.

RAW ONIONS FOR *RAJAS*

The kinetic quality of our universe, *rajas*, is always moving. Foods that are stimulating to the senses increase rajas, the mobile quality of mind and body. When I eat raw onion, I am distracted by the strong taste in my mouth for the rest of the day and sometimes longer. In the next morning's yoga practice, I smell onion in my sweat. Being followed around by the smell of something eaten yesterday suggests the far-reaching effect of rajas. Foods that are fresh, whole, and energizing but not stimulating are called *sattvic*. Their mellow flavors increase feelings of quietude, comfort, and well-being, and nourish the body without exciting the mind or senses. This cilantro-mint chutney is a great example.

summer ayurvedic spice mix

You will notice the other seasonal chapters feature a salt recipe. Here I've eliminated it because the humidity of summer warrants a lower salt intake. Rejoice in the tastiness of fresh herbs instead of salt (see the sidebar "Fresh Herbs" for an easy tip)—you will reduce water retention and the puffy or bloated feeling some folks get in the heart of summer. Cardamom and turmeric counteract stomach acid, so integrating the Summer Spice Mix into your meals will balance a potential increase of hot, sharp qualities.

SUMMER SPICE MIX

1 tbsp whole coriander seeds

1 tbsp whole cumin seeds

1 tbsp whole fennel seeds

1 tbsp turmeric powder

½ tsp cardamom powder

Dry roast the coriander, cumin, and fennel seeds in a heavy-bottomed pan on medium heat for a few minutes, until you can smell them. Let them cool completely. Grind to a uniform consistency in a spice-dedicated coffee grinder or by hand with a mortar and pestle. Transfer to a small bowl and stir in turmeric and cardamom powders until well combined. Store in an airtight jar or shaker top container.

FRESH HERBS

In lieu of a recipe for a seasonal salt, here's a tip for keeping fresh herbs around the kitchen in a form that can be added quickly to any of your summer and fall soups and spreadables.

Herbed Ice Cubes

Buy one or two bunches of fresh parsley, cilantro, or basil—or better yet, grow them! Soak the herbs in water to remove dirt, then shake off excess water and press with a clean towel to dry. Pull the leaves off the stems with your fingers or chop them off with a knife and discard the stems. (The stems of most herbs are too bitter for eating.) Set aside a big handful of leaves to be used the same day for garnish to a dish or as an ingredient in a summer recipe. Then, in blender carafe or food processor, process the rest of the leaves with enough water to make a thick puree. Pour into ice cube trays and freeze. You now have fresh-frozen herb cubes that can be added to juices, soups, chutneys, and sauces in a jiffy.

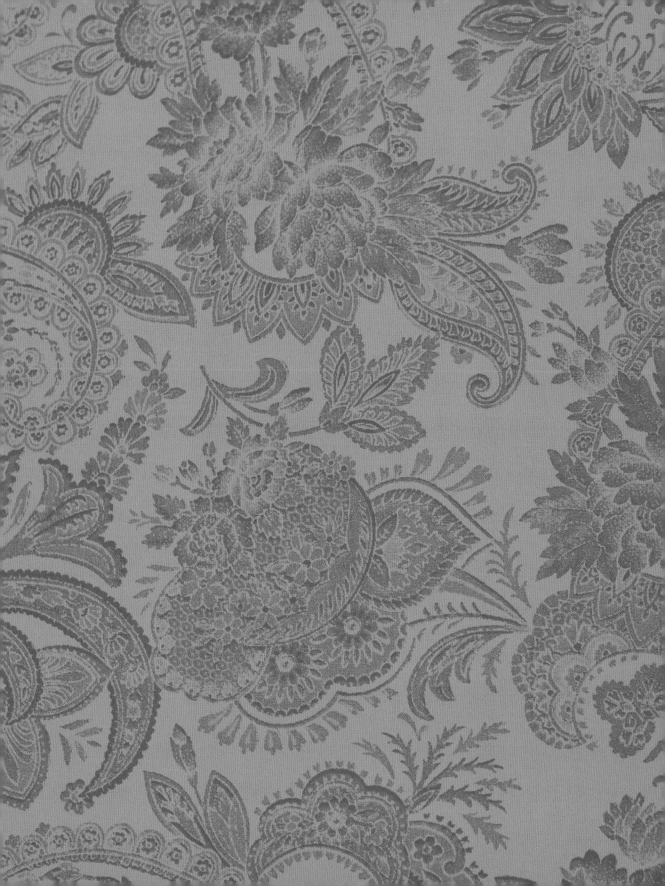

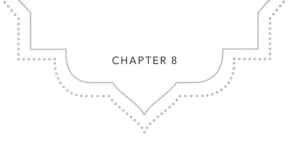

CHAPTER 8

Fall Recipes

BUILDING FOODS TO TRANSITION THROUGH COOL, CRISP, CHANGEABLE WEATHER

The leaves are beginning to change color and the air is light, crisp, and clear. Fall winds stir up the landscape, signaling the coming of cooler weather. This is an important time to prepare the body for the cold months by clearing out accumulated summer heat and storing nourishment in the deep tissue layers to sustain energy through the winter. Cooking with the early fall harvest of bitter and astringent foods such as cranberries, dark leafy greens, and pumpkins helps the body expel leftover heat. As the appetite grows and temperatures drop, cravings for sweet, moist foods are fed by these recipes that feature builders like coconut oil, figs, sesame seeds, and oats.

Fall Diet and Lifestyle Overview

The Elements: Air and ether; fire (early fall)
Feels Like: Cool, dry, rough, windy, light

QUALITIES TO INTRODUCE	QUALITIES TO REDUCE
Warming	Cold
Grounding	Mobile (doing too much)
Moist	Dry
Rhythm, routine	Erratic lifestyle

POTENTIAL SIGNS AND SYMPTOMS OF IMBALANCE	TASTES TO ENJOY
Gas, bloating, and constipation	Sweet
Dry skin and scalp	Bitter and astringent (early fall)
Anxiety	Salty and sour (late fall)

Fall Foods Guide

Favor warm, moist, slightly oily, and building foods.

FOODS TO FAVOR

- Root vegetables, such as sweet potatoes, carrots, turnips, parsnips, beets, and winter squashes
- Cooked cold-weather greens, such as sea vegetables, collards, kale, and Swiss chard
- Warming spices, such as cinnamon, ginger, cumin, fennel, and salt
- Warm, spiced cow's, almond, or goat's milk; diluted yogurt
- Raw or fresh-roasted seeds and nuts
- Rich cold-pressed oils, such as coconut or sesame; ghee; avocados
- Moist grains, such as wheat, brown rice, and oats, cooked with a little extra water
- Sweet or heavy fruits, such as bananas and mangos; apples, pears, and cranberries (early fall)
- Proteins from small legumes, such as red lentils, mung beans, split peas, and adzuki beans; tofu; eggs; most meats for nonvegetarians

FOODS TO REDUCE

- Dry foods, such as chips and crackers
- Coffee and other forms of caffeine
- Carbonated drinks, including bubbly or seltzer water
- Large beans (cannellini, kidney, pinto), which may cause wind
- Raw foods

FALL LIFESTYLE GUIDELINES

- Use a warm, medium-bodied oil, such as almond or sunflower, for your morning massage. Use sesame oil if you feel cold and dry. You may add woody, grounding essential oils, such as sage and cedar.
- Consume warm food and drinks. Avoid skipping meals, and do not fast.
- Establish regular mealtimes.
- Keep your ears covered in the wind and cold.
- Wear warmer clothing as the temperature drops.
- Stay hydrated by drinking warm water.
- If you suffer from allergies or worry about coming down with the flu, practice neti and nasya daily.
- Take care to relax, get enough rest, and nap if needed.

FALL SHOPPING LIST

VEGETABLES	FRUITS	GRAINS	FATS	SPICES
Beets	Apples	Brown rice	Avocados	Cardamom
Broccoli	Bananas	Oats (rolled	Coconut,	Cloves
Carrots	Cranberries	and steel cut)	shredded	
Collards	Dates	Red rice	Coconut milk	EXTRAS
Kale	Figs	Wheat berries	Cow's milk	Cacao powder
Parsnips	Pears		Eggs	Coconut sugar
Pumpkins	Raisins	BEANS	Goat's milk	Maple syrup
Spinach		Black beans	Raw nut butters	Nasya oil
Squashes			Raw nuts	Sesame oil for
Swiss chard			Tahini	massage
Turnips				

fig cardamom oat cup

serves 1

On days when having breakfast to go is unavoidable, this oat cup can be made ahead of time, allowing the oats and dried fruits to soak up the almond milk. The stable, grounding nature of almonds and oats will balance the erratic, mobile qualities that can arise when you're on the go. Take care to keep your cup out of the refrigerator so it is at room temperature when you eat it. On a cold day, add a bit of ginger tea from your thermos to create a hot breakfast when the time comes to sit quietly and enjoy it.

BREAKFAST

⅓ cup rolled oats

3 dried figs, quartered

1 tsp maple syrup

⅛ tsp ground cardamom

½ cup almond milk

Combine all the ingredients in a clean half-pint (8-ounce) glass jar, adding almond milk last. Seal with a lid and shake to combine. Let the mixture soak at room temperature for a few hours before eating or keep it in the fridge overnight and toss it in your bag the next morning for a destination breakfast.

NOTE: For a late fall option, add grated apple, substitute molasses for the maple syrup, and replace the cardamom with apple pie spice.

EATING ON THE GO

If, once in a while, you find yourself without even ten minutes to sit down and have breakfast, you will need nourishment while on the move. I'm including a few to-go recipes to help you continue to eat home cooking even when things get busy. But remember, eating on the go is not a sustainable way of life. Create good food options as often as you can, and stay focused on bringing a busy phase back into balance by knowing that eating well supports you in your healthy path and keeps you feeling good.

One important caution: eating in a moving vehicle, such as a car, train, or plane, is not recommended in any season, as the mobile quality will disturb the digestion and, when repeated habitually, can result in discomforts like acid stomach, gas, bloating, or constipation. If eating in a vehicle is unavoidable, mindfully notice your situation: take a few deep breaths first, slow the mind, relax the belly, and welcome the food in with full attention. Eat especially slowly. At these times, consuming less complex foods and ones that require less chewing than your normal meals means less bloating or belching. See Spiced Nut Milk Smoothie for one such recipe (page 235).

SEASONAL RECIPES AND ROUTINES

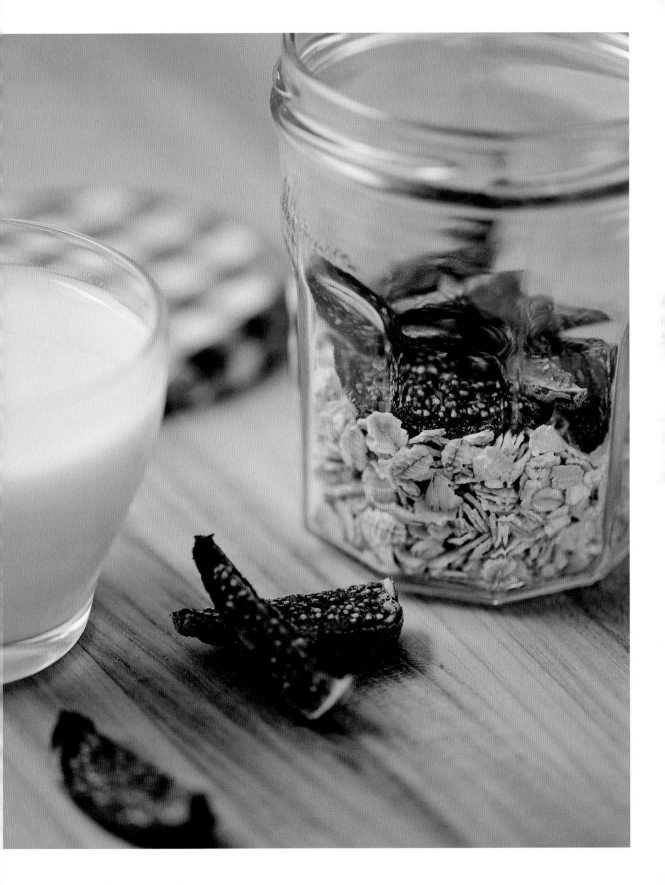

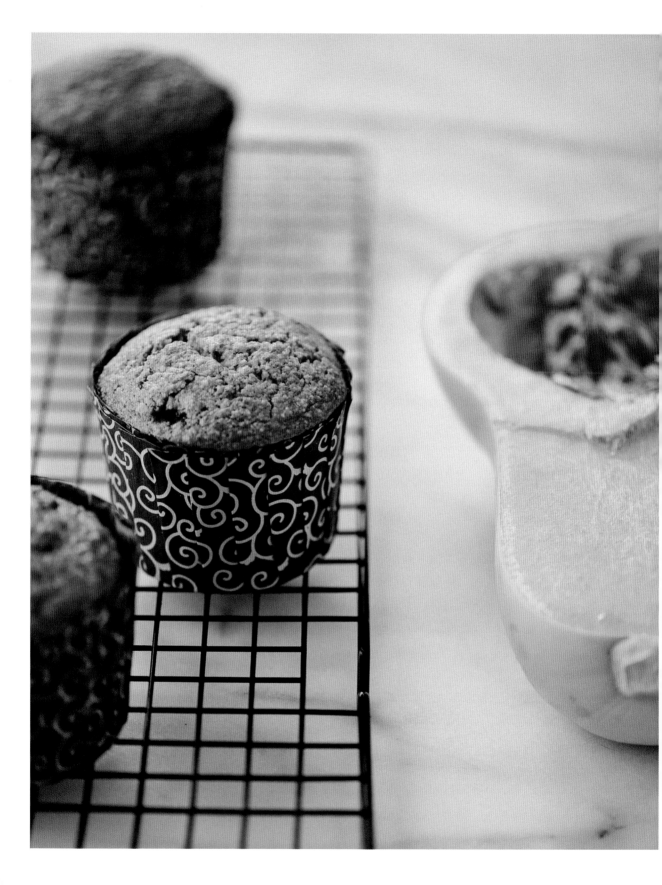

cranberry butternut muffins

makes 6

Fall's dry, light, windy days will make you crave heavy, grounding foods like winter squash and nuts, and these muffins deliver deep nourishment. This is a grain-free, high-protein recipe that features cooked squash and almond meal as the bulk of the muffin. The drying astringency of both squash and cranberries is balanced by moist, natural fats and sweet, warming spices for a complete breakfast. (Author's note: These muffins received a messy thumbs-up from photographer Cara's toddler, Evelyn.)

2   eggs (or substitute 2 flax "eggs"—see below)
½   cup cooked butternut squash
¼   cup maple syrup
2   tbsp coconut oil, melted
1½ cups almond meal
¼   tsp salt
¼   tsp baking soda
¼   tsp baking powder
1–2 tsp Everyday Sweet Spice Mix (see page 118)
¼   fresh cranberries, chopped
2   tbsp shredded coconut

Preheat oven to 350 degrees. Line muffin tins with baking cups.

In a medium-size mixing bowl, whisk the eggs briskly with a fork for 1-2 minutes. Add the squash and mash into the egg. Stir in the maple syrup and melted coconut oil.

In a separate small bowl, mix together the almond meal, salt, baking soda, baking powder, and spice mix. Add the dry ingredients to the wet and stir together. Do not overmix. Stir in the cranberries.

Divide the batter into 6 muffin cups. Dust with the shredded coconut. Bake for 25 minutes or until tops begin to brown. The muffins will be soft and will firm up as they cool. Let muffins cool completely before removing from tins.

To make 2 flax "eggs": In a blender carafe, combine 2 tbsp ground flaxseeds and 6 tbsp water; blend on high speed for 2 minutes. Substitute for eggs in the recipe.

stewed apples with dates

serves 2

When you don't have a big appetite or a lot of time, this quick compote is both handy and healing. Raw apples can be too cool, hard, and rough to eat raw in the fall. Cooking apples balances their cold quality, making this light but satisfying compote ideal for early fall. Apples will remove residual summer heat from the body when served warm and moist, with sweet dates. The benefits of apple's cooling, cleansing qualities are many.

BREAKFAST

2 apples, cored and chopped
4 dates, pitted and cut in half
2 cups water
1 tbsp maple syrup
1 tbsp grated fresh gingerroot (optional)
1 tsp Everyday Sweet Spice Mix (see page 118)

In a small saucepan or frying pan, combine the chopped apples and dates, water, maple syrup, and spices. Bring to a boil over high heat, then turn down to medium-low and simmer for 5 minutes. Remove from heat and blend with an immersion hand blender for just a few seconds, maintaining a chunky consistency, or process about one-third of the mixture in a blender carafe until smooth and stir it back into the saucepan with the chunky fruit.

To serve, divide into 2 breakfast bowls.

NOTE: You can substitute raisins, dried prunes, or apricots for dates; like apples, all these fruits also contain the cleansing cool of astringent taste. Raisins and prunes especially are lighter than dates and indicated for weight loss.

SEASONAL RECIPES AND ROUTINES

fall roasted spiced vegetables with whipped tahini sauce

serves 4

Root vegetables are naturally sweet and have building, rejuvenating qualities. Pair them with ghee or coconut oil, and you have an excellent tonic to prepare your body for winter. Chop, toss, and roast, and a glorious tray of food emerges from your oven. You can roast most hearty vegetables and toss them with herbs like marjoram and thyme. This recipe is my favorite mixture of root vegetables that cook at a similar rate. Note: the smaller you cube the vegetables, the faster they cook. (I generally dice them into minute, half-inch cubes in hopes of eating in thirty minutes!) Always cut vegetables into uniform-sized pieces to ensure even roasting.

FALL ROASTED SPICED VEGETABLES

2 medium beets, peeled
2 carrots
2 parsnips
2 medium yams or ½ butternut squash, peeled
2 tbsp ghee or coconut oil
1 tbsp tamari (optional)
1 tbsp chopped fresh rosemary, fennel seeds, or Fall Spice Mix (see page 240)

Preheat the oven to 375 degrees. Chop all of the vegetables into roughly ½-inch cubes.

Put the ghee or coconut oil into a small, oven-safe dish and place it in the oven for 1–2 minutes, long enough to melt the fat. Use an oven mitt or pot holder to remove the container from the oven.

In a large bowl, toss the cubed vegetables together with the melted ghee or oil, tamari, and rosemary, fennel seeds, or spice mix until all the cubes are evenly coated. Spread them in a single layer on the bottom of a large 9 x 13-inch baking dish. Bake for 20 minutes. Remove the pan from the oven and turn the vegetables over with a spatula. Bake 10–20 minutes more, until the vegetables are soft; some pieces will begin to brown. Remove from the oven, toss on the tray, and serve immediately with a side of Whipped Tahini Sauce for dipping.

Roasted vegetables are also quite festive served with Cranberry Clove Chutney (page 241).

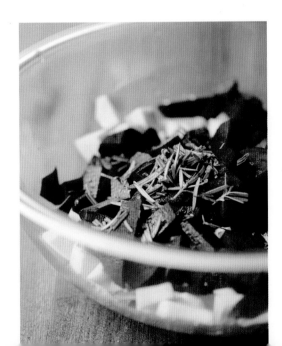

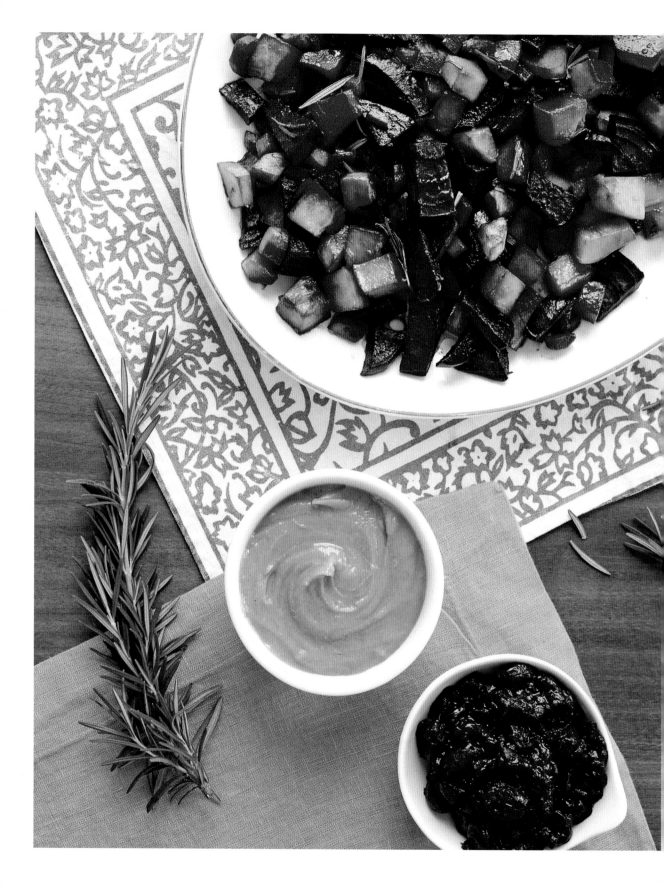

WHIPPED TAHINI SAUCE

Tahini, or sesame butter, is to me the most delicious way to reap the benefits of sesame's deeply nourishing and moisturizing effects. This seed is an ojas-building tonic full of iron and protein. If you have a light, dry body, Whipped Tahini Sauce can be a staple year-round.

This sauce can be made to order—whip it right in the serving bowl with a fork and voilà! The recipe makes a thick sauce for dipping hot roasted root vegetables. Anytime you need a rich topping for your grains or other vegetables, add a bit more water and process in a blender to make a creamy dressing.

½ cup tahini

2 tbsp olive oil

juice of ½ lemon

½ tsp salt

Put the tahini in a bowl large enough for you to whisk all the ingredients. (Rather than coating a measuring cup with messy sesame butter, make an educated guess and spoon the tahini directly into the mixing bowl. A slightly interpretive measurement will not ruin your end product.) Add oil, lemon juice, and salt. Whip briskly with a fork or whisk. There will be a moment when the oils begin to separate—keep whipping! The mixture will become smooth. Add water, 2 tbsp at a time, if you'd prefer to pour the sauce rather than spoon it.

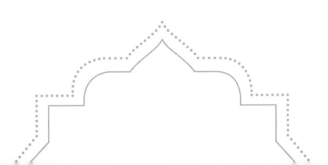

red pumpkin dal

serves 4

Red lentils cook up quickly, are easy to find in most stores, and are light, dry, and slightly heating. The sweet, oily qualities of coconut milk balance the dry qualities of lentils and astringent squash. This thick, gravylike dal is excellent served over light and fluffy basmati rice. I often serve this one for guests, because it is consistently quick, filling, and delicious.

LUNCH

4 cups water or 3 cups water plus one 16-oz can coconut milk

1 cup red lentils

1 tsp Fall Spice Mix (see page 240)

1 tsp dehydrated sugarcane or maple syrup (optional)

1 small *kabocha* squash (about 2 cups chopped)

½ tsp salt

TEMPERING

1 tbsp coconut oil

1 tsp grated fresh ginger

½ tsp cumin seeds

½ tsp mustard seeds

2 tbsp shredded coconut

Boil the water and coconut milk, if using, in a large saucepan on high heat. Rinse the red lentils until the water runs clear. Add lentils to the boiling water along with the spice mix and sweetener. Allow to come to a boil again, uncovered. Then turn heat down to medium.

Chop the squash, peel and all, into 1-inch cubes. Add to the saucepan. When it boils again, turn heat down to low and simmer, partially covered, for 30 minutes. Do not stir.

Heat the oil in a small frying pan on medium heat and temper the ginger, cumin seeds, and mustard seeds until you smell them, just 2–3 minutes. Take the pan off the heat and stir the shredded coconut into the hot pan. Continue to stir for a minute or two as the coconut browns.

Add this tempering to the lentils and squash, along with the salt. Simmer the dal, uncovered, for 5 minutes more.

Serve as a soup or ladle over rice.

NOTE: Kabocha skin, unlike butternut or acorn squash, gets completely soft when cooked and adds green color to the dish. I would much rather eat it than peel it, but it works both ways if you would like to cut the peel off before cubing.

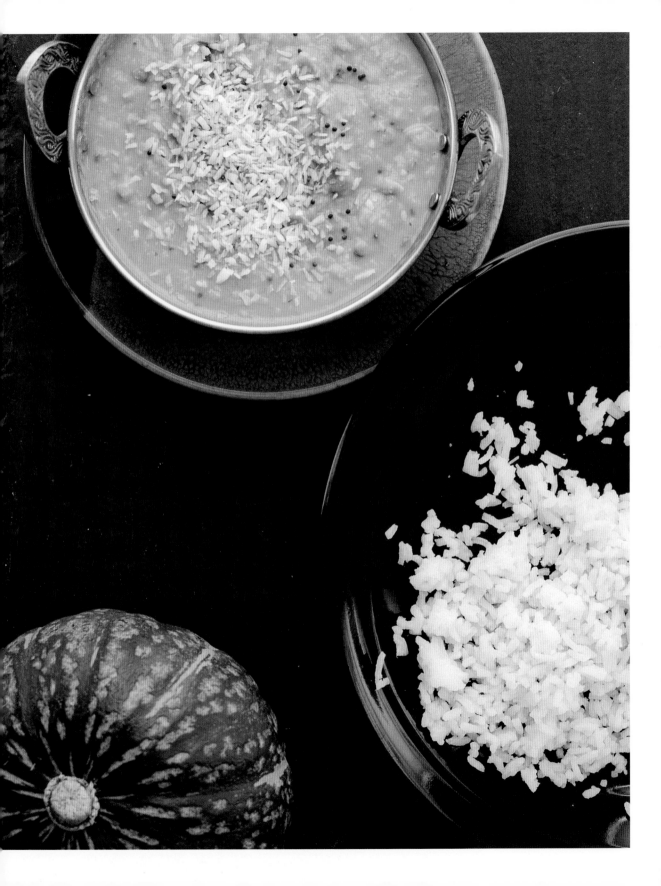

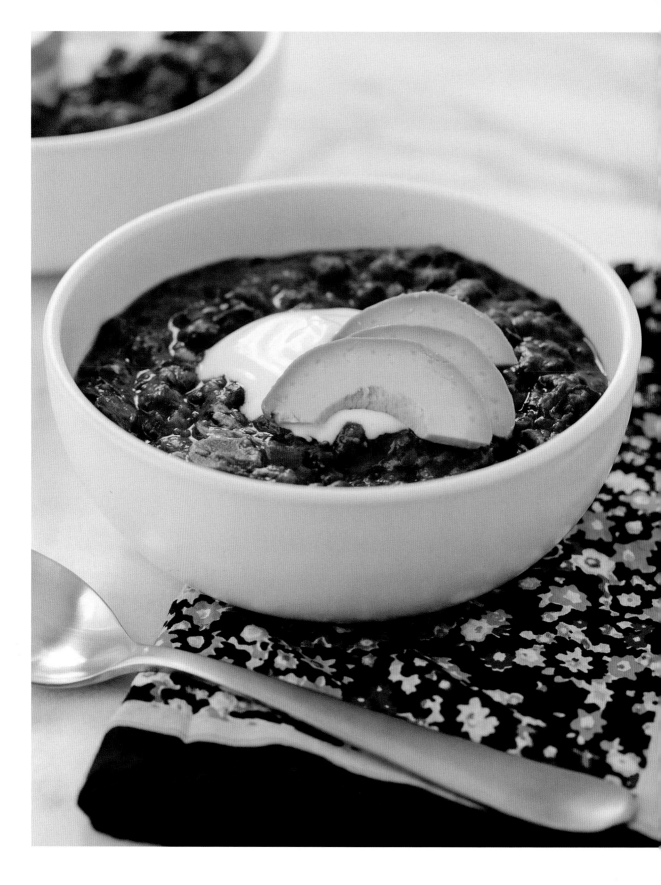

simple black bean soup

serves 4

In Ayurveda, beans are known to nourish superficial as well as deep tissue layers, especially the muscle tissue, which makes them a strong addition to a vegetarian diet. Cumin and coriander stoke the digestive fire, and beans are always prepared with digestive spices in Ayurvedic cooking. Serve this thick soup over a cooked grain, with a sprouted grain tortilla or dosa—or you may find it is filling enough on its own.

3 cups cooked black beans

1½ cups cooking water from the beans or vegetable broth

2 large carrots, chopped

2 large leaves Swiss chard, chopped

1 tsp turmeric powder

1 tbsp ghee

1½ tsp cumin seeds

1 tsp coriander powder

½ tsp salt

OPTIONAL GARNISHES
(choose one):

sliced avocado

chopped fresh cilantro

fresh tomato (in moderation), chopped

dollop of yogurt

In a large saucepan, bring the beans, water or broth, vegetables, and turmeric powder to a boil over high heat. Cover and simmer on low heat for 15-20 minutes, until vegetables are soft.

While the beans and veggies are cooking, warm the ghee in a small frying pan over medium heat. Add the cumin seeds and sauté until you can smell them, just 2-3 minutes. Remove them from the heat right away. Add the seasoned ghee and coriander powder to the pot with the beans and continue to simmer 5 minutes more. Remove from heat and stir in salt.

Use an immersion hand blender to process the soup to the desired consistency. Blending only about half of the beans and vegetables will give your soup a creamy base with a hearty texture.

Serve in a bowl with avocado slices, diced tomato, or a dollop of fresh, whole milk yogurt and sprinkle with chopped cilantro.

NOTE: If you have trouble with gas when you eat beans, cook them a very long time, until the beans begin to break apart. Because the beans are blended up in this soup, the skins will be easier to digest than if they were whole.

quick dal saag

serves 4

Supercleansing. Supereasy. Supersatisfying. The spice mix in this recipe brings a grounding dose of sweet and salt tastes to a bitter and astringent pairing. While traveling in India, I've often found that spinach dal is the only green food available for months, and this dish has become dear to my heart. I have simplified the recipe so you too can make this one a staple dish, without needing to buy a long list of ingredients or using an overload of garlic and onion.

• • • • •

1 cup split yellow mung beans

4 cups water or broth

1 tbsp Fall Spice Mix (see page 240)

1 tsp turmeric powder

3 oz baby spinach, roughly chopped

½ tsp salt

4 tsp melted ghee for garnish

Soak the split mung beans in water for at least 3 hours or overnight. Rinse the mung beans until the water runs clear.

In a large saucepan, bring the 4 cups of water or broth to a boil over high heat. Add the mung beans, spice mix, and turmeric to the saucepan and bring back to a boil, uncovered. Turn the heat down to medium and simmer without stirring, partially covered, for 20 minutes (at least 30 minutes if you did not soak the mung beans first). Stir in the chopped spinach until it wilts. Add salt.

Serve in 4 bowls over brown or white basmati rice or with Everyday Dosa (see page 97). Garnish each serving with 1 tsp melted ghee.

NOTE: If you want to go the extra mile, temper 1 tsp mustard and cumin seeds in 2 tsp ghee until you can smell the spices, then stir into the dal near the end of the cooking time. As for the spinach, organic baby spinach is so easy to cook with and widely available, there is little need to use frozen spinach. The vitality of fresh food cannot be under-estimated . . . but if you must use frozen spinach, this recipe will require only 3 cups water. Watch out for the Ayurveda Police, however, and use it at your own risk!

the yam bomb

serves 2

This recipe is not for the faint of appetite. Yams do not have the dry quality of squash and are purely sweet, warming, and building—a good choice when they are in season. Eat them in moderation if you are trying to lose weight, however. Make a quick dinner by putting the yams in the oven right when you get home from work. Take some time to relax or unpack the day's bag while they cook. You may interchange sweet potatoes and yams.

2 medium-size yams

2 tsp ghee, coconut oil, maple syrup, and/or almond butter

Everyday Sweet Spice Mix (see page 118) or cinnamon to taste

Preheat the oven to 350 degrees. Poke each yam with a fork a few times. Place on a baking sheet or in a baking dish and bake until the yams are completely cooked through, about 30 minutes or more, depending on how fat the yams are. Pierce the skin with a fork to see if the flesh inside is soft, and when it is, remove the yams from the oven and cut an X in the tops. Peel back the skin and press the sides of each yam to create a hollow pool.

To serve, fill each pool with 1 tsp each ghee, coconut oil, maple syrup, and/or almond butter. Sprinkle with Everyday Sweet Spice Mix or cinnamon to taste. Whipped Tahini Sauce (see page 217) is also delicious to dress a savory bomb. Eat with a steak knife and fork.

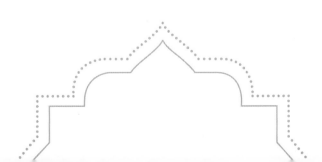

raw beet slaw with lemon and mint

serves 4

The power of the beet cannot be underestimated, especially in the fall. Beets are bitter, astringent, and sweet. They clean the blood and the bile ducts of accumulated summer heat, and speed up the elimination channels that expel it. A serving of this slaw a few times per week will keep the doctor away. Or, to get the cleansing benefits of beets without the extra preparations, simply squeeze fresh lemon juice on shredded beets and serve as a side dish.

1 large or 2 small beets, peeled and grated

juice of ¼ lemon

1 mint sprig (optional)

1 tbsp sunflower seeds

salt to taste

Mix grated beets and lemon juice together in a small bowl. If using mint, tear the leaves into small pieces by hand or snip with kitchen shears and add to the beet mixture.

In a small frying pan, toast the sunflower seeds on low heat for about 5 minutes, until lightly browned, gently shaking the pan or stirring as needed to keep the seeds from burning.

Add the sunflower seeds and salt to the beet mixture and stir again.

Serve ½ cup pile beside tofu tacos or inside a collard wrap. This also makes a great side dish to serve beside Everyday Cleansing Green Soup or Everyday Kichari.

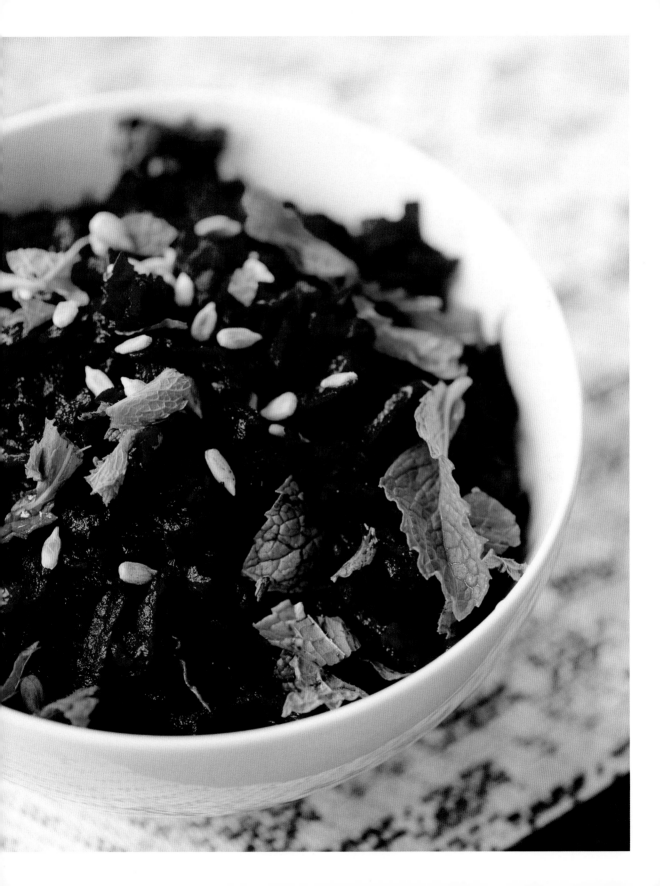

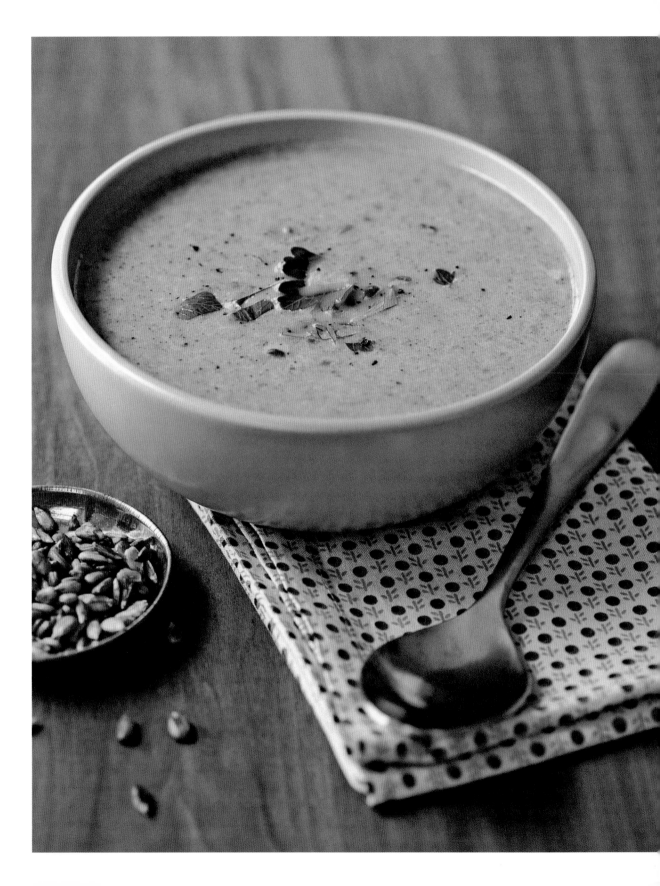

surprising cream of broccoli soup

serves 2

Surprise! Broccoli's gentle bitterness and goat milk's sweet creaminess make an amazing soup! On a cold day, trust me, it's delicious. While developing the Everyday Cream of Anything Soup recipe, we stumbled onto this inspired pairing. Goat's milk is easy on the gut because it has a warming effect and is lighter than cow's milk, thanks to its pungent *vipak*, or postdigestive effect. This means your body can break down the fat well, and the milk will nourish your deep tissues.

SUPPER

2 cups diced broccoli florets
and stems

2 cups vegetable broth

½ cup goat's milk

½ cup chopped fresh parsley
(optional)

½ tsp salt

pepper to taste

In a medium saucepan, boil the broccoli in the broth until tender, about 10 minutes. Please note that the smaller you dice up the stalks, the faster they will cook and the more easily your body will digest them. Remove from heat and add the milk, chopped parsley, and salt. With an immersion hand blender, process to a smooth consistency. Divide into 2 bowls and sprinkle with fresh ground pepper.

WHY GOAT'S MILK?

Ayurveda takes into account the postdigestive effects of all foods, or the action the food has on the body, called *vipak*. For instance, gingerroot tastes pungent on the tongue, but the aftereffect on the body has the qualities of sweet taste—building and cooling—as opposed to the pungent qualities of hot and light.

Both cow's and goat's milk are heavy and oily, both taste sweet on the tongue, but they have very different postdigestive effects on the body. Unlike cow's milk, which has a sweet vipak to encourage building and grounding qualities, goat's milk has a pungent vipak to encourage lightening and warming qualities. The pungent vipak makes goat's milk lighter on the digestion than cow's milk. The changes of season, namely spring and fall, can be a difficult time to digest heavy foods, and goat's milk delivers some fats and proteins in an easier-to-digest form.

FALL RECIPES

coconut buttercup soup
with ume pumpkin seeds

serves 4

Ayurveda uses harmonious food combinations to encourage a harmonious body and mind. Not only do coconut and this exceptionally sweet squash taste perfect together, they also have complementary qualities: dry squash meets oily coconut and cooling squash meets warming spices to create a balanced dish. When the bright orange skin of the buttercup squash shows up at the fall farmers' market, I am sure to make this soup within the week.

SUPPER

COCONUT BUTTERCUP SOUP

1 medium-size buttercup squash
1 12-oz can coconut milk (1½ cups)
2 cups water
1 tsp cinnamon
¼ tsp nutmeg
½ tsp salt

Preheat oven to 350 degrees. Cut the squash in half, scoop out the seeds, and place each half facedown in a 9 x 13-inch glass baking dish with 1 inch of water. Bake until the squash is completely soft and yields easily to a fork inserted into the skin, about 30 minutes. Remove from the oven and place the halves on a plate to cool slightly.

Warm the coconut milk and water in a large saucepan over medium heat. Scoop out the flesh of the squash with a large spoon and stir in to the saucepan along with the cinnamon, nutmeg, and salt. Bring all to a boil, lower the heat, and simmer for 5 minutes. Remove from heat and, using an immersion hand blender, process the mixture until smooth and creamy.

Serve in 4 wide bowls, sprinkled with Ume Pumpkin Seeds.

UME PUMPKIN SEEDS

Ume plum vinegar, a Japanese condiment, is unique in that it has the properties of all three building tastes: sour, sweet, and salty. This vinegar makes an exciting cool weather condiment.

½ cup raw pumpkin seeds
½ tsp ume plum vinegar

Spread the pumpkin seeds in a heavy-bottomed pan and toast for about 5 minutes on the stove top over low-medium heat. Stir the seeds or shake the pan every minute or so. Once the seeds start to pop, stir and toast them for 1 minute longer, then remove from heat. Transfer the seeds into a wide dish to cool for a few minutes. Dash the ume plum vinegar on top and toss to distribute.

Serve as garnish on a soup or have a handful as a snack.

SEASONAL RECIPES AND ROUTINES

kate's apple crisp

serves 4-6

This recipe represents two of the best things about autumn: local apples and baking. Friends have been known to show up at the house with a peck of apples and a hopeful grin. I invite them in and preheat the oven. Making crisp with friends is a great activity while catching up. One can prepare the apples while another makes the crisp.

Without flour or sugar, Kate's Apple Crisp contains only a few whole, easy-to-digest ingredients. The cooling effects of apples and coconut, along with the astringency of cranberries, make for an excellent early fall treat to cool down the system. Jonagolds are my favorite type of apple for crisp.

4 medium-size apples, chopped (about 5 cups)

juice of ½ small lemon

1 tsp Everyday Sweet Spice Mix (see page 118)

2 tbsp raisins

2 tbsp dried cranberries

¾ cup oats

¾ cup almond meal

3 tbsp coconut oil, melted

3 tbsp maple syrup

¼ tsp salt

¼ cup shredded coconut or chopped walnuts (optional)

Preheat the oven to 375 degrees.

In a large mixing bowl, toss together the apples, lemon juice, spice mix, and dried fruits.

Make the topping in a separate mixing bowl, using a fork to stir together the oats, almond meal, coconut oil, maple syrup, salt, and shredded coconut or walnuts, if using.

Transfer the tossed apple mixture into an 8 x 8-inch glass baking dish. Distribute the topping in a layer over the apples and pat down gently with your hand. Cover the pan with foil and bake for 40 minutes, or until apples are bubbling and soft. Take the pan from the oven and remove the foil, then bake uncovered for 10 more minutes, or until topping is crisp.

Use a large spoon to transfer hot crisp into dessert bowls.

NOTE: There are as many crisps as there are bakers! Some recipes have as much topping as they have apple; others blend berries, pears, or chopped nuts with the apples. I swear by coconut oil instead of butter, and the almond meal is my secret ingredient. These easy-to-digest fats and proteins transform the traditional crisp into a complete meal. I love to serve it with a dollop of yogurt on the side.

baked apples

serves 4

Baking these apples will make your home smell like the holidays. This recipe is worth the effort—baking apples renders them very digestible and cleansing. The slow, steady heat of baking increases the grounding quality of the otherwise light and dry apple. Because they take a little time, it's nice to bake them up in a batch and plan to warm up a leftover apple for another meal the next day. Taking a baked apple to enjoy at work will bring you that cozy feeling.

¼ cup dried cranberries

½ cup raisins

4 dried figs, finely chopped

2 dried apricots or pitted dates, finely chopped

3 tsp Everyday Sweet Spice Mix (see page 118)

1 cup apple juice, cider, or water

4 large apples

16 whole cloves

4 tsp honey for garnish (optional)

Preheat oven to 350 degrees.

Mix the dried fruits, spice mix, and liquid together in a small bowl and let them soak while you core the apples (see sidebar "Apple Coring 101"). Pierce each apple with four cloves (for flavor and decoration). Place the apples side by side in an 8 x 8-inch baking dish. Spoon the filling into the cored apples, letting some sit on top of the apples. Pour remaining juices over their tops and into the baking dish. Bake 25 minutes, or until very tender. For added flavor, partway through baking you can baste the apples by spooning some of the liquid from the bottom of the pan over them. Remove from the oven and let them stand for 5 minutes.

To serve, drizzle 1 tsp of honey over the top of each apple, if you like. Eat with a steak knife and fork.

NOTE: If you tend toward gas when you mix fruit with other food, resist the temptation to have these for dessert and enjoy them instead at breakfast time, when the stomach is empty, or as a light supper on their own.

APPLE CORING 101

To core the apples if you don't own an apple corer, send a paring knife straight down into the apple alongside the core and parallel to the stem, keeping the skin on the bottom intact. Do this three more times, creating a square around the core. The square should be big enough to surround the seeds. Dig out the bottom of the square with the knife tip and pull the core out of the apple by its stem. Check to make sure you caught all the seeds.

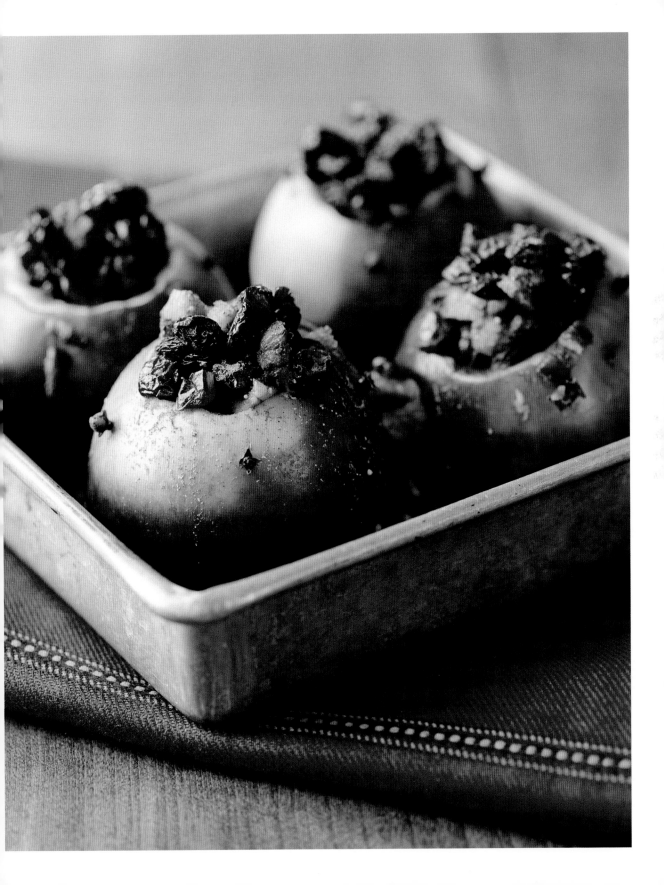

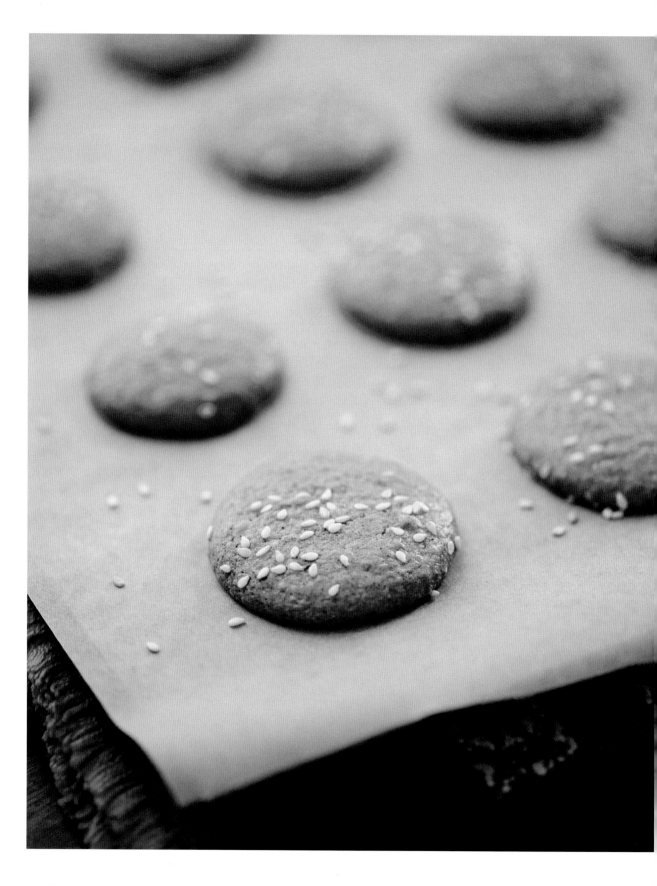

sesame cookies

makes 2 dozen

Sesame is a rainy-season crop, revered in Ayurveda as an ojas builder and often used for making sweets in the winter season and for devotional festivals. Sesame is special because it contains an unusual trio of tastes: bitter, pungent, and sweet. Its naturally balanced composition of heating, cooling, and building qualities makes it a tonic for increasing strength and immunity. Note: This cookie should retain a chewy inside.

1 cup sesame tahini

¼ cup almond flour

⅓ cup maple syrup

½ tsp pure vanilla extract

2 tsp Everyday Sweet Spice Mix (see page 118)

¼ tsp salt

½ tsp baking soda

1 egg, whisked (or substitute 1 flax "egg"—see below)

2 tsp sesame seeds, plus extra for decoration

Preheat oven to 350 degrees. Prepare 2 baking sheets by lightly greasing with ghee or coconut oil or else lining with parchment paper.

In a medium mixing bowl, mix the ingredients together in the order listed. If the batter is too runny to shape, put it in the fridge for 5–10 minutes (but batter that's a little runny bakes nicely). Shape batter into tablespoon-size balls or drop with a spoon onto the prepared cookie sheets. Leave a few inches between the balls, as they will puff up when they bake. Lightly press down on the balls with a fork. Sprinkle tops with extra sesame seeds. Bake for 10–12 minutes, until they are firm enough to touch without your finger sticking.

Let them cool completely before removing from baking sheets and serving. Puffs will be soft when you eat them.

To make 1 flax "egg": In a blender carafe, combine 1 tbsp ground flaxseeds with 3 tbsp water and blend on high for 2 minutes.

VARIATION: PEANUT BUTTER TRUFFLE COOKIES

Only at Christmastime, I make these with peanut butter in place of tahini, omit the spices and almond flour, and stir in chocolate chips to make a flourless truffle cookie. Because the peanut butter is thicker than tahini, the batter will be thick enough to drop onto the cookie sheets without any almond flour. The result is a smooth, melt-in-your-mouth experience. Very decadent—one is enough!

pumpkin chia pudding

serves 2 for dessert or 1 for an entrée

This pudding will make you want to curl up and hold your cup close. Pumpkin is cooling in nature and astringent, making it one of those fall foods that cool and tone the gut after a humid summer.

· · ● ● ● · ·

2 tbsp chia seeds

½ cup almond milk

½ cup pumpkin puree

½ tsp vanilla

1 Medjool date or 2 soaked deglet moor dates, pitted

1 tsp maple syrup or molasses

1 tsp Everyday Sweet Spice Mix (see page 118) or pumpkin pie spice

dash of freshly grated nutmeg

In a small bowl, soak the chia seeds in the almond milk for 5 minutes, whipping with a fork a few times to evenly distribute.

Put the pumpkin, the vanilla, dates, maple syrup or molasses, and spice mix into a blender carafe. Add the chia mixture on top. Blend on high speed for 2 minutes, creating a smooth, whipped texture. The chia seeds and dates should disappear into the puree.

Divide into 2 dessert goblets or eat it all from a big bowl as a main meal. A dash of freshly grated nutmeg on top makes this pudding very special.

BAKING SUGAR PUMPKINS

Using canned pumpkin is easy, but so is baking small, sweet pumpkins—and once you've tried both, the difference in taste is hard to ignore. When little sugar pumpkins are available in the fall, buy a few—the smaller they are, the sweeter they will be. Cut them in half, scoop out the seeds, and place them facedown in a baking dish in about an inch of water. Bake at 350 degrees until soft, about 30 minutes. Once they have cooled, scoop out the flesh and put it in a glass storage container for mixing into cereals, baked goods, and puddings.

spiced nut milk smoothie

serves 1

Spiced Nut Milk Smoothie is a great aftermeal treat and also a complete breakfast in a jar. Use warm water, a pint-size mason jar, and a hand blender. You can drink it right up or take it to go. By not straining out the pulp, as you would when making almond milk, you'll get a little thicker and more filling drink. If your system is sensitive to fiber and you tend to experience bloating, soaking and skinning the almonds ahead of time will solve that problem.

¼ cup almonds, soaked
   (see "Kitchen Techniques,"
   page 302)

¾ cup warm water

1 tsp maple syrup

¾ tsp Everyday Sweet Spice Mix
   (see page 118)

½ tsp pure vanilla extract
   (optional)

pinch of salt

Place the soaked almonds and ¼ cup of the warm water in a pint-size wide-mouth glass mason jar. Using a hand blender, process to a smooth paste. Add the remaining ½ cup warm water, maple syrup, spice mix, vanilla extract, if using, and salt. Blend until smooth. Drink immediately.

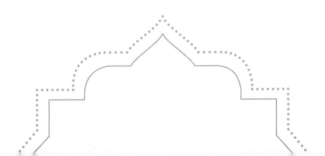

fall digestive tea

serves 2

Licorice root, an herb, counteracts the dry quality of fall with its demulcent quality—an ability to aid the body in holding water in the intestines. This herb, called *yashtimadhu* in Sanskrit, is widely used to lubricate the intestines, much like slippery elm and marshmallow root. Fennel reduces leftover summer acidity, while cinnamon and ginger warm the gut.

2 cups water
¼-inch piece fresh gingerroot
½ tsp fennel seeds
½ tsp cinnamon
1 tsp licorice root powder or
    2 tsp chopped licorice root

In a small saucepan, bring 2 cups of water to a boil.

Coarsely chop the gingerroot—don't worry about removing the skin. Add the chopped ginger, fennel seeds, cinnamon, and licorice powder or pieces to the water. Reduce heat to low and simmer, covered, for 10-15 minutes.

Pour through a small tea strainer into 2 mugs to serve. Take 6 ounces with or after meals.

WHY PRACTICE ABHYANGA?

A great way to manage the dry quality of fall is the practice of abhyanga, an Ayurvedic oil massage in which one stimulates the circulation by rubbing the skin with oil in a specific pattern and direction. According to the Ashtanga Hridayam, "Abhyanga should be resorted to daily, it wards off old age, exertion and aggravation of vata; bestows good vision, nourishment to the body, long life, good and strong, healthy skin."[1] This is a valuable aspect of the Ayurvedic practice, especially during the cold and dry seasons.

Stress Reduction

Review "Artha: Misuse of the Sense Organs" (page 24) to understand how your skin, eyes, ears, nose, and tongue are a direct line to your nervous system. The skin is the largest of your sensory organs, and it is exposed to the qualities and energies of your environment all the time. Oiling the skin creates a subtle protective layer around your body and your energy field.

Circulation

In order for the body to deliver nutrients, hormones, and sensory information where they need to go and to eliminate what has to go out, circulation must be strong and consistent. For best results, make sure that your strokes as you apply oil are firm and stimulating, yet calm and rhythmic.

Practicing self-massage stimulates the circulation, and encourages the smooth flow of prana. See Seasonal Self-Care 1 (page 288) to learn how to practice oil massage.

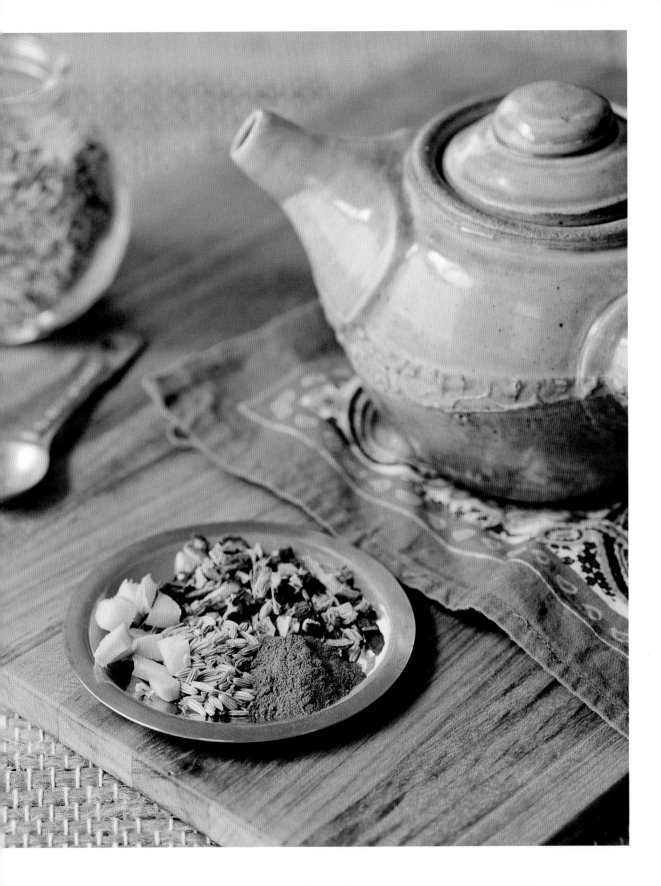

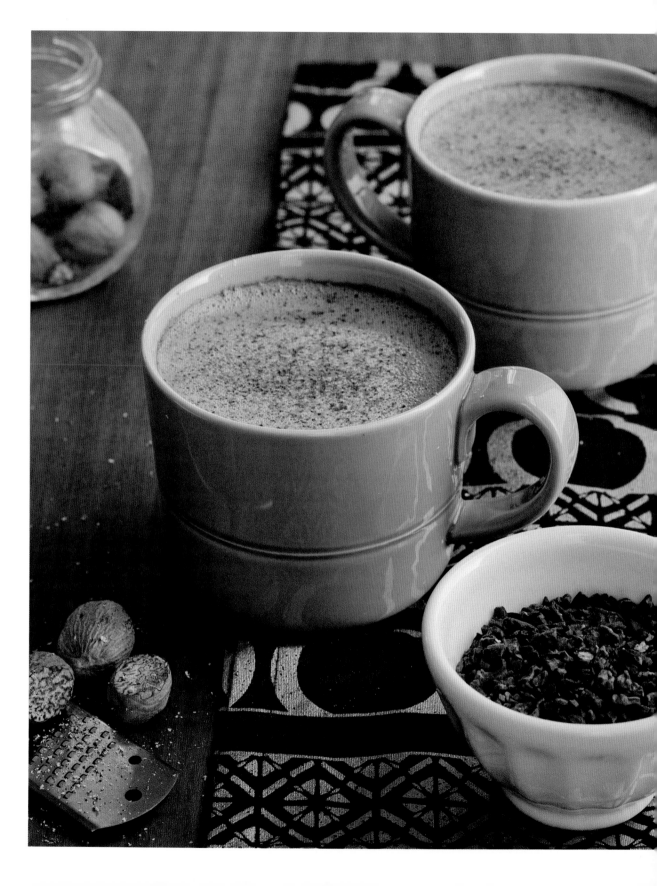

medicinal hot cocoa

serves 2

This cocoa is made medicinal with the addition of ashwagandha. Sometimes known as Indian ginseng, the plant's root is used for its restorative benefits, nourishing the bone layer and strengthening the immune system, as well as supporting sexual potency. Use of this herb keeps the body strong like a horse, for which the herb is named (*ashwin* means "horse"). The addition of ashwagandha to hot cocoa makes it thicker, malty tasting, and darned good for you, too—but if you don't have it, you can still make this hot cocoa. Due to its heating energy, ashwagandha is generally recommended for use only in cold weather.

2 cups almond, sunflower, or cow's milk

1 tbsp maple syrup, coconut sugar, or raw cane sugar

¼ cup cacao powder

1 tsp cinnamon or Everyday Sweet Spice Mix (see page 118)

1 tsp ashwagandha

2 cinnamon sticks or freshly grated nutmeg for garnish (optional)

Begin to warm the milk in a medium saucepan on medium heat. Add the sweetener and the cacao powder. Whisk briskly until it begins to steam. Take off the heat and whisk in the cinnamon or spice mix and ashwagandha by hand or use a hand blender. I am a staunch believer in the smooth texture and cappuccinolike foam that results from a 30-second churn with the hand blender.

To serve, pour into 2 mugs. Care to impress guests? Grate fresh nutmeg atop the foam or serve each cup with a cinnamon stick.

COCOA OR CACAO?

Where you put your a's and o's makes a big difference. The processing of cacao into cocoa renders it a denatured food; in other words, the food has come a long way from its birth as a cacao pod, using lots of resources for its travel, absorbing energies from its time spent in factories and packaging. To make your own whole-food, low-impact cacao, I recommend buying raw cacao nibs and grinding up a jar's worth in a coffee grinder on your day off. Take your time to grind it to a very fine powder. The bags of cacao powder are nice, too, but will cost you more than grinding the same amount yourself.

fall ayurvedic spice mix and salts

A shake of the Fall Spice Mix in your cooking will create a balancing effect, aiding the digestion in shifting from hot to cool weather. Balance the cool, dry, light qualities of the season by choosing warm, moist, well-spiced (but not hot and spicy) dishes. The Fall Spice Mix encourages strong digestive fire and stimulates and soothes the digestive organs. When you aren't in the mood for Indian flavors, the Fall Salts will bring stimulating, fresh tastes from the herb garden to your cooking. A dry fall day deserves a bit more salt, while a wet one needs less.

EXTRAS

FALL SPICE MIX

makes ¼ cup

1 tbsp coriander seeds
1 tbsp cumin seeds
2 tsp fennel seeds
1 tbsp turmeric powder
2 tsp ginger powder

Dry roast the coriander, cumin, and fennel seeds in a heavy-bottomed pan on medium-low heat until you can smell them, a few minutes. Transfer the seeds from the pan to a wide bowl and cool completely. Grind the whole roasted seeds to a uniform consistency in a coffee grinder dedicated to spices or by hand with a mortar and pestle. Pour them back into the bowl and stir in the turmeric and ginger powders.

Store in a small jar with an airtight lid or in a glass spice jar with a shaker top. This recipe makes about a month's supply.

FALL SALTS

makes ¼ cup

1 tbsp sage
1 tbsp rosemary
1 tbsp thyme
1 tbsp sea salt
1½ tsp black pepper

Grind the herbs in a mortar and pestle until fine enough to fit through your shaker holes.

Mix the dried herbs, salt, and pepper together in a glass shaker jar. These salts can be used in cooking and also kept on the table as a condiment. Makes about a one-month supply.

cranberry clove chutney

makes 16 ounces

Cranberries' punch can focus your energy, and the berries cleanse the blood and digestive organs with their powerful combination of astringent and sour tastes: sharp and penetrating, yet cooling. Cranberry Clove Chutney will keep you feeling sharp and energized while aiding your digestion of heavy foods. Making this chutney will save you the extra sugar of store-bought cranberry sauce.

1   lb fresh cranberries
2   cloves
1   tsp cinnamon
¼-inch piece gingerroot,
    peeled and finely chopped
    or grated
1   cup orange juice
1   tbsp orange zest
½   cup dehydrated cane juice

In a medium saucepan, combine the cranberries, spices, ginger, orange juice, and orange zest. Bring to a boil over high heat. Turn the heat down to low and stir in the dehydrated cane juice. Simmer all the ingredients together, uncovered, until the cranberries begin to dissolve and the chutney clings to a spoon, about 20 minutes. The chutney will thicken a bit more as it cools.

You can cut back on the sweetener in this recipe, adding it only to taste, but it will need to cook 5–10 minutes longer to thicken.

Serve a tablespoon with steamed kale, roasted vegetables, or cream of grain cereal.

LATE FALL VARIATION: Add 6 black peppercorns to the mix for increased warmth.

CLOVE ATTACK!

The cloves can stay in the chutney to further infuse, but watch out when you are dishing it out! To tell the truth, I remove them before storing the chutney, because I find biting into a clove really unpleasant. I have bitten into many a strange spice pod in my travels, and when I am cooking at home, I try to avoid such adventures.

gingered apple butter

serves 6

This versatile spread harmonizes well served with squash, cooked in oatmeal, or spread on muffins. Adding fresh ginger to the recipe makes the butter a digestive addition to main meals and baked goods. Although Ayurveda normally recommends not mixing fruit with other foods (see "Mixing Fruits with Other Food," page 45), cooking the apples makes combining them acceptable.

6 apples, cored and coarsely chopped

¼ cup apple cider or apple juice

1 tbsp maple syrup

¼-inch slice fresh gingerroot, peeled and coarsely chopped

1 tsp Everyday Sweet Spice Mix (see page 118)

In a medium-size saucepan, combine the chopped apples, apple cider or apple juice, and maple syrup. Heat on medium-low heat, adding the chopped gingerroot and spice mix while it warms. Simmer 30 minutes. Take off the heat. Blend with a hand blender or food processor to a smooth puree. Cool and store in a pint-size mason jar. Spread on muffins or top creamed grain cereal.

To make Pear Butter, substitute 3 cored, chopped pears for 3 of the apples.

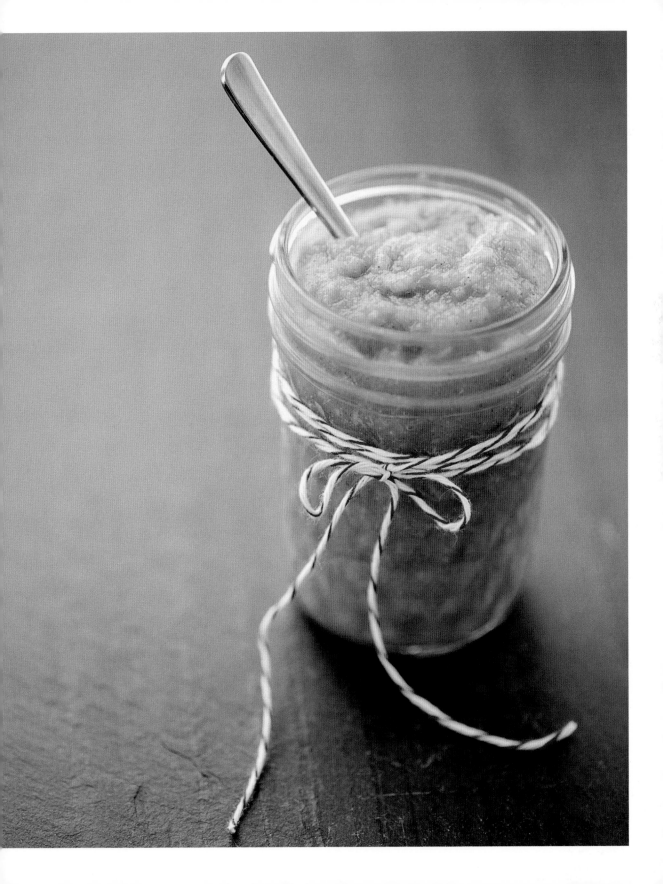

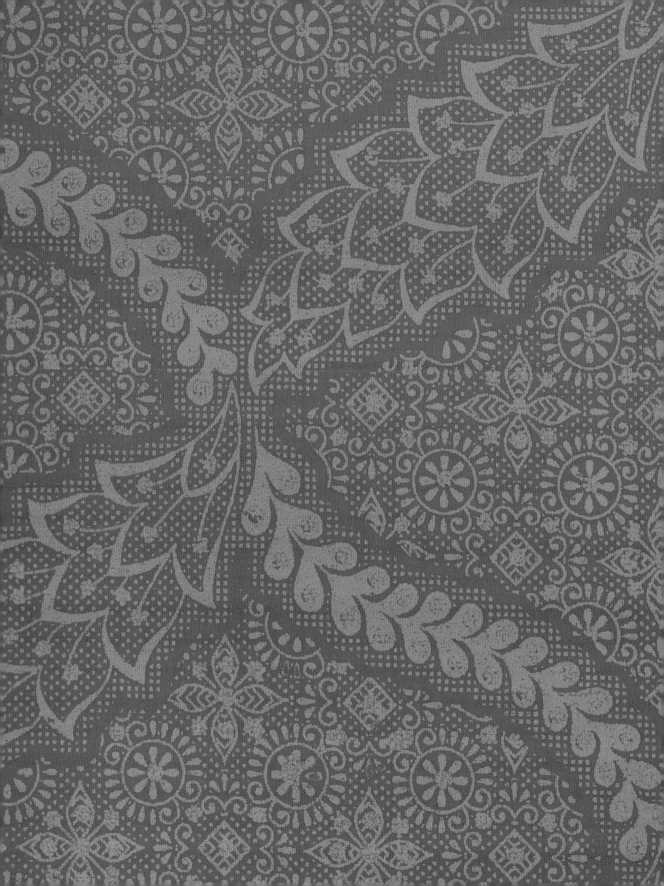

CHAPTER 9

Winter Recipes

MEALS TO NOURISH AND GROUND THE BODY IN COLD, DRY SEASONS

The air is dry, cold, clear, and light. Gentle morning dew hardens into snow and ice. Most vegetation is storing energy in its roots, protected from the season's cold, rough winds. Our bodies do the same, and we put on hats, gloves, and boots to keep the extremities warm. The digestive fires naturally accumulate in the core in cold weather, and the body's furnace is at its best to digest and metabolize delicious winter recipes of healthy fats and proteins. Ayurveda suggests enjoying the hearty, dense, and oily qualities of foods like nuts, sweet potatoes, and ghee. The following nicely spiced, warming, grounding recipes feature such ingredients as dates, sprouted beans, cooked fruits, and cinnamon. Use the winter recipe section to keep you feeling centered and burning bright.

Winter Diet and Lifestyle Overview

The Elements: Air and ether
Feels Like: Cold, dry (especially inside when the heat is on), light, windy, rough, hard

QUALITIES TO INTRODUCE/REDUCE

Introduce	*Reduce*
Warming	Cold
Moist	Dry
Grounding	Erratic
Soft	Hard

POTENTIAL SIGNS AND SYMPTOMS OF IMBALANCE

Constipation
Dry, cracking skin and joints
Cold hands and feet
Weight gain
Lethargy and sadness

TASTES TO ENJOY

Sweet
Sour
Salty

Winter Foods Guide

Favor cooked, protein-rich meals, including soups and stews.

FOODS TO FAVOR

- Starchy vegetables, such as sweet potatoes, root vegetables, and squash; cold weather greens, such as sea vegetables, kale, collards, and chard; artichokes (late winter). Be sure to take bitter taste in moderation—it makes you cold—and balance bitter greens with sweet grains or root vegetables.
- Warming spices, such as cinnamon, ginger, cumin, salt, black pepper, chilies, and vinegars (in moderation); unrefined sweeteners such as maple syrup, raw honey, and molasses
- Warm, spiced almond, cow's, or goat's milk; diluted yogurt
- Raw or home-roasted seeds and nuts; nut butters
- Rich oils, such as ghee and sesame
- Moist grains, such as wheat, brown rice, and oats, cooked with a little extra water
- Sweet or heavy fruits that bring moisture and building qualities, such

as oranges, bananas, dates, figs, papayas, mangoes; grapefruits and lemons (very good in late winter)
- Proteins, such as lentils, small beans, tofu, and eggs; most meats, for nonvegetarians; winter is the season for occasional red meat if you eat it.

FOODS TO REDUCE
- Dry foods, such as chips and crackers
- Raw foods
- Drying grains, such as millet, rye, and barley
- Cold foods, especially dairy products
- Fruits and vegetables that are not in season

WINTER LIFESTYLE GUIDELINES
- Use a rich, warm oil, such as sesame, for your morning massage. You can add sweet, warming scents, such as sweet orange and rose oils, to the sesame. Be sure to massage the oil into the scalp at least once a week and wash your hair after one hour or the following morning.
- Wear a hat and scarf to protect the ears and neck from accumulating cold and hard qualities.
- Practice nasya (oiling the nose) in the morning or at bedtime (see page 291). Use a humidifier in your bedroom at night.
- Take moderate exercise daily, such as yoga, dancing, and walking.
- Wear colors and keep colorful things around you.
- Sit in a steam room or take warm baths at least once a week.

WINTER SHOPPING LIST

VEGETABLES
Artichokes
Beets
Carrots
Collards
Kale
Parsnips
Roasted red
 pepper (once or
 twice a month)
Sea vegetables
 (dulse, nori,
 wakame, sea
 palm)
Squashes
Sweet potatoes
Swiss chard
Tomatoes,
 farm-canned
White potatoes,
 in moderation
Yams

FRUITS
Apples
Bananas
Dates
Grapefruit
Mangoes (ripe for
 eating and green
 for chutney)
Oranges
Papayas
Pears

GRAINS
Brown rice
Bulgur wheat
Oats
Red rice
Rice noodles

BEANS
Black beans
Green lentils
Red lentils

FATS
Almond butter,
 raw
Almond meal
Cashews
Coconut,
 shredded
Cow's milk
Eggs
Goat's milk
Sesame oil
Sunflower butter
Tahini

SPICES
Chili powder
Paprika
Red chilies, dried

EXTRAS
Apple cider
Cacao powder
Maple syrup
Molasses
Rice vinegar

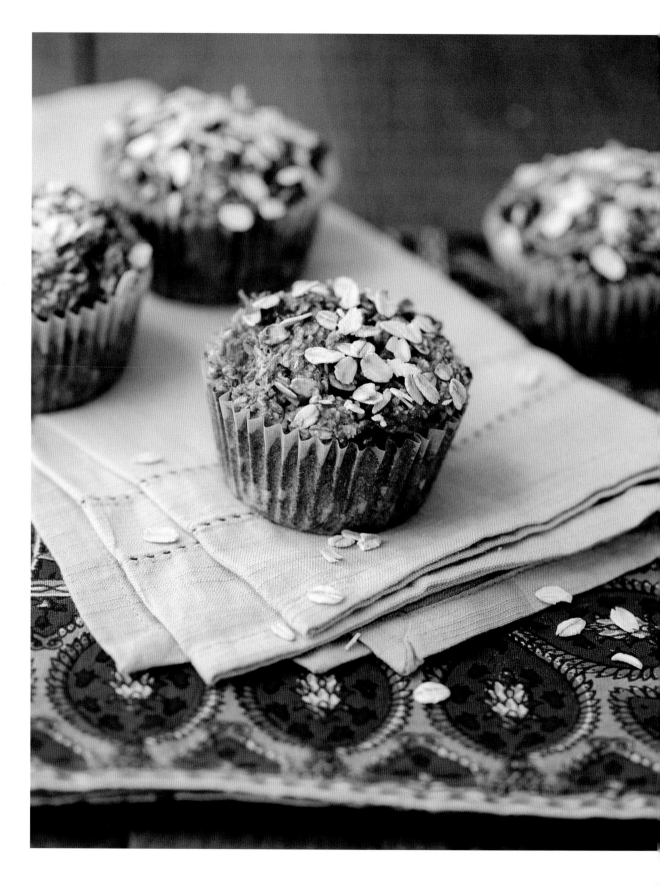

yam and oat muffins

makes 6

The yam (or sweet potato) is a vegetarian's best friend. Pair it with the minerals found in molasses, and this recipe will provide a goldmine of building qualities to help you recover after working out, to warm you up when you get home, to feed a sweet tooth, and to nourish people you love—especially you. The recipe contains no oil, so be sure to spread each muffin with ghee, coconut oil, or nut butter. You can also pair these muffins with Gingered Apple Butter (page 242).

1 egg (or substitute 1 flax "egg"—see below)

½ cup whole cow's milk or almond milk

½ cup mashed sweet potato

1 tbsp maple syrup or molasses

½ cup oats (to grind)

½ cup rolled oats

¼ tsp baking soda

⅛ tsp baking powder

¼ tsp cinnamon

¼ tsp ginger powder

⅛ tsp nutmeg

pinch of salt

1–2 tsp ghee, coconut oil, or nut butter per muffin, for garnish

MIX-INS (OPTIONAL):

½ cup chopped pecans

¼ cup chopped pitted dates

Preheat the oven to 400 degrees. Line muffin tin with muffin cup liners or grease the muffin tin with coconut oil.

In a small mixing bowl, whisk the egg until fluffy, then stir in milk, mashed sweet potato, and maple syrup or molasses.

To grind ½ cup of oats, place oats in dry blender carafe or food processor and pulse until ground. This will take less than a minute. In a large mixing bowl, mix the ground oats together with the rest of the dry ingredients.

Stir the wet ingredients into the dry ingredients, just enough to incorporate. Do not overmix. Gently fold in your optional mix-ins. Evenly distribute batter into 6 cups. Bake for 30 minutes, or until tops are golden and a toothpick inserted in muffin center comes out clean.

Serve each muffin spread with 1–2 tsp of ghee, coconut oil, or nut butter to provide the oils needed in winter.

To make 1 flax "egg": In a blender carafe, combine 1 tbsp ground flaxseeds with 3 tbsp water and blend on high for 2 minutes.

IS THAT A YAM?

Sweet potatoes and yams are used interchangeably in Ayurvedic recipes, but they are not quite the same vegetable. Sweet potatoes have brown skin, orange flesh, and the richer vitamin content of the two. Yams are purple skinned, and have pale flesh. Yams are larger, sweeter, and have a milder flavor than sweet potatoes. I often choose sweet potatoes for soups because of their bright color, yet in these muffins, yams taste sweeter.

overnight bulgur wheat breakfast

serves 2

Bulgur can cook overnight by soaking it in hot water. Just warm it up in the morning and add some vegetables to the same pot for a hearty, savory, one-pot meal. You can grate or shred vegetables in advance (it only takes a minute in a food processor) and keep them in an airtight container in the fridge. When you add them in the morning, they will cook in a few minutes. A savory breakfast, as opposed to a sweet one, sets you up for a steady day. Take the leftovers for lunch and serve with a Black Bean and Oat Burger (see page 256) or a Red Lentil Pâté and Mineral Gomasio (see page 267, 265).

BREAKFAST

1 cup bulgur wheat

2 cups boiling water or vegetable broth

2 tsp Winter Spice Mix (see page 283)

¼ cup raisins or ½ cup grated carrots or yams or shredded cabbage (optional)

pinch of salt

Rinse the bulgur wheat and place in a medium saucepan. Pour 2 cups boiling water or broth over the grains, cover, and soak overnight.

In the morning, add Winter Spice Mix and a bit of water to the pan to keep the bulgur wheat from sticking to the bottom and turn the heat up to medium. Add raisins, if using, or vegetables. (You can grate the carrots or yams or shred the cabbage right into the pot, if you like.) Do not stir. Cover and steam for 7–10 minutes.

Add salt and fluff with a fork before serving in 2 bowls.

NOTE: You can make this recipe without vegetables; soak the raisins and the spice mix overnight with the bulgur wheat and simply warm the cereal on the stove top for a few minutes before eating.

ghee fried apples

serves 1

Reminiscent of pie, but without the crust, this warm breakfast takes only a few minutes to prepare and satisfies a light appetite.

· ● ● ● ● ·

2 tsp ghee

½ tsp Everyday Sweet Spice Mix (see page 118)

1 large apple, cored and sliced

1 tbsp raisins or chopped figs (optional)

Warm the ghee and spice mix in a small frying pan on medium heat. Add the apple slices to the pan and stir to coat all the pieces. Fry on medium heat for 2-3 minutes, stirring. Add a tablespoon or two of water to keep the apples from sticking to the pan, and fry for 2-3 minutes more, until tender.

For variety, add raisins or chopped figs with the water.

Transfer to a small bowl and enjoy as is.

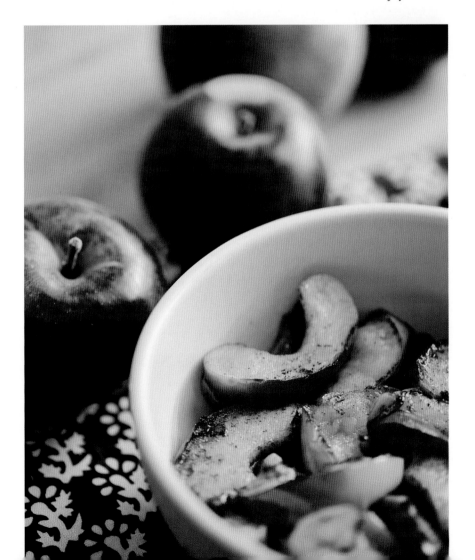

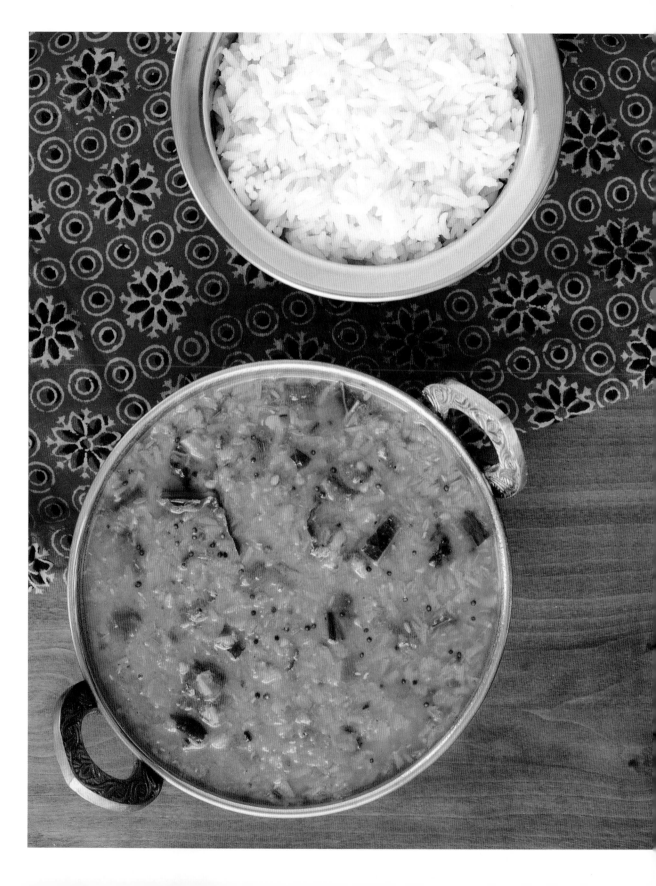

warming tomato dal

serves 4

While red lentils and tomatoes together are primarily a heating combo, this dish also satisfies the pungent, sour qualities we crave in winter. The bright colors—yellow, green, and red—are a welcome sight in deep winter. Balance the heating qualities of the dal by serving it over a sweet grain, such as basmati rice, or with a sprouted wheat tortilla.

....●●●●●..

4   cups water

1   cup red lentils

1   tbsp Winter Spice Mix (see page 283)

2   whole fresh tomatoes or one 16-oz can whole tomatoes, chopped (reserve juice)

2   leaves lacinato kale

1   tbsp ghee

½   tsp cumin seeds

½   tsp black mustard seeds

1   tsp salt

In a large saucepan, bring the 4 cups of water to a boil over high heat. Rinse the lentils until the water runs clear. Add the lentils to the water along with the spice mix.

In a separate, small pot, parboil the whole fresh tomatoes, stem and all, in water for 4–5 minutes. Pull out with a slotted spoon and cool them until you can slide the skins off. Discard the skins, coarsely chop the tomatoes, and add to the dal. If you are using canned tomatoes, add the tomatoes and their juice to the dal. Bring to a boil again, then turn heat down to low and simmer, uncovered. Set a timer for 30 minutes, then slice the kale leaves into thin ribbons and add to the pot. Continue to simmer, partially covered, until the timer hits 30 minutes.

Let the dal simmer on low while you warm the ghee in a small frying pan over medium heat and sauté the cumin and mustard seeds until you can smell them, just 2–3 minutes. If the mustard seeds are jumping out, cover the pan.

Add the spiced ghee and the salt to the lentils and boil, uncovered, 5 minutes more.

Stir and serve in 4 wide bowls with rice or tortillas.

NOTE: This recipe also works great in a slow cooker or pressure cooker. Red lentils don't need to be soaked overnight, although any dal will be creamier if you do soak the legumes.

TOMATO TALK

Tomato skins are difficult for some people to digest and contain more acid than the inside of the tomato—making skins a potential irritant. Parboiling tomatoes to remove their skins is the traditional method in India, where there are many tomato dishes. One cannot digest so many tomato skins in a day. Removal of skin creates a milder dish, one that's easier on the gut and also nicer to look at, as there will be no floating pieces of skin.

Canned tomatoes, though convenient, will not have the vitality of fresh ones. However, if you put the energy into growing and canning your own, you are likely to feel great eating them, thanks to the prana and sattva fresh food provides.

black bean and oat burger

serves 2

This easy recipe can be doubled, and you will have extra patties to pack for tomorrow's lunch. A Black Bean and Oat Burger served over an Everyday Steamed Salad Bowl or paired with rice and mango chutney will keep you warm any winter day.

LUNCH

1 cup cooked black beans
1 handful baby spinach
¼ cup diced roasted red pepper
⅓ cup oat flour (see below)
1 tsp Winter Salts
1 tsp ghee (optional, for frying)

Preheat oven to 350 degrees. Line a baking sheet with parchment paper.

In a large mixing bowl, mash the beans well with a fork. Continue to mash in all the other ingredients except the ghee until the mixture reaches a uniform but chunky consistency. Form 2 large or 3 medium-size patties, lay them on the parchment paper, and bake for 10 minutes on each side. Alternatively, you can melt 1 tsp of ghee in a frying pan and pan fry the burgers slowly over medium heat, about 5–7 minutes on each side, until well browned.

TO MAKE OAT FLOUR: pulse rolled oats in a blender carafe until finely ground.

NOTE: If you don't suffer from any signs of internal heat (see "Understanding Internal Climate," page 68), you can substitute salsa for the roasted peppers.

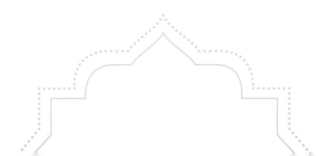

huevos rancheros and brussels sprouts hash

serves 2

This is one of those complicated recipes for a fun brunch or just for you when you have the time and a hankerin' for a special meal! Traditional huevos rancheros can be a food-combining nightmare, but fear not—I have applied Ayurveda's helpful hints to the creation of this warming dish. For protein, choose either eggs or beans and serve with Brussels Sprouts Hash on the side. To keep preparation simple, omit the ranchero sauce and serve just the eggs or beans with hash.

RANCHERO SAUCE

NOTE: Since this recipe requires a bit of work, it makes 4 servings. Keep the extra 2 servings to eat with grains or vegetables later.

½ cup diced red onion

½ clove garlic, diced (optional)

2 tsp ghee

1 tsp chili powder

1 tsp cumin powder

1 tsp coriander powder

1 heaping tsp paprika

dash of cayenne powder

½ tsp salt

1 cup chopped tomatoes

1 cup chopped celery

1 cup chopped carrots

1 cup vegetable broth

In a medium-size saucepan or large frying pan, fry the onions and garlic, if using, in the ghee over medium heat, stirring, until they soften, a few minutes. Add the spices and stir. Then add the tomato, celery, and carrots, stirring for 1 minute more. Pour in the broth and simmer, uncovered, for 30 minutes. Take off the heat and process with an immersion hand blender just long enough to make a chunky sauce. Cover to keep warm.

BRUSSELS SPROUTS HASH

2 cups Brussels sprouts

1 tbsp ghee

dash of salt

Shred the Brussels sprouts by holding on to the stems and grating with the large holes on a box grater, or cut off the stems and pulse in the food processor.

Warm 1 tbsp ghee in a large frying pan, then add the shredded Brussels sprouts, stirring. Add a dash of salt and continue stirring. Remove from heat when hash is browned to your taste. Spread the corn tortillas over the hash and cover to warm while you make the eggs.

HUEVOS (OR BEANS) RANCHEROS

4 eggs or 1 cup cooked
   black beans
1 tsp ghee
1 tsp turmeric powder
   (for eggs)
4 corn tortillas
chopped fresh cilantro
   (optional)

If using eggs, warm the ghee in a large frying pan, break the eggs directly into the pan, and sprinkle with turmeric. Fry the eggs until the yolks just begin to harden. If using cooked beans instead, warm them in a saucepan with 1 tsp ghee and mash with a fork or, for a creamy texture, process with a hand blender.

TO SERVE

Place 2 warm tortillas on each plate. Divide the eggs or beans into 2 servings over the tortillas. Spoon Ranchero Sauce on top. Divide the Brussels Sprouts Hash and serve beside the tortillas. Garnish with chopped fresh cilantro, if desired.

NOTE: If you do not own 2 large frying pans, use a smaller one for the hash and warm the tortillas in the oven. Preheat to 275 and spread the tortillas on a baking sheet. Remove when warm, after 3-5 minutes.

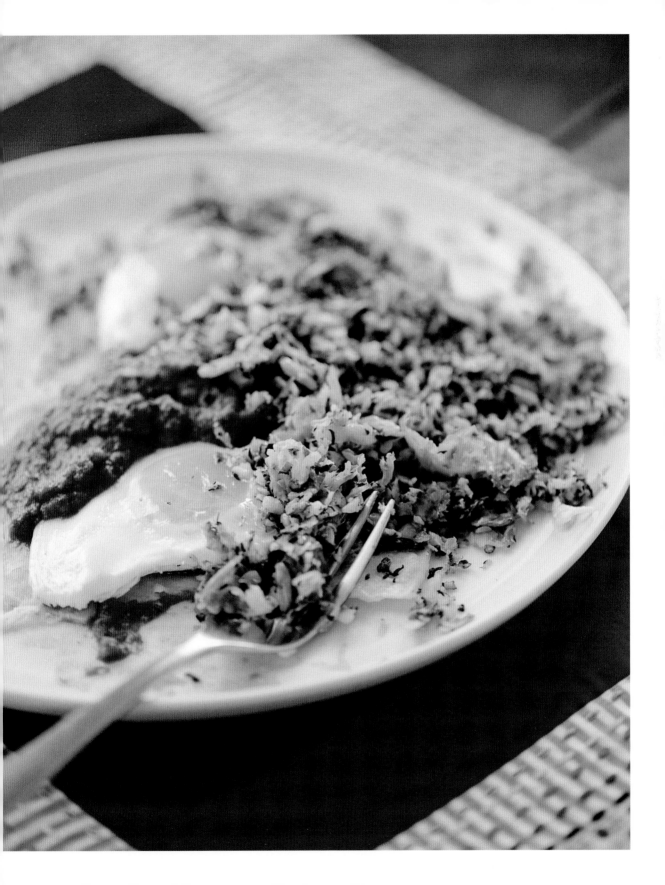

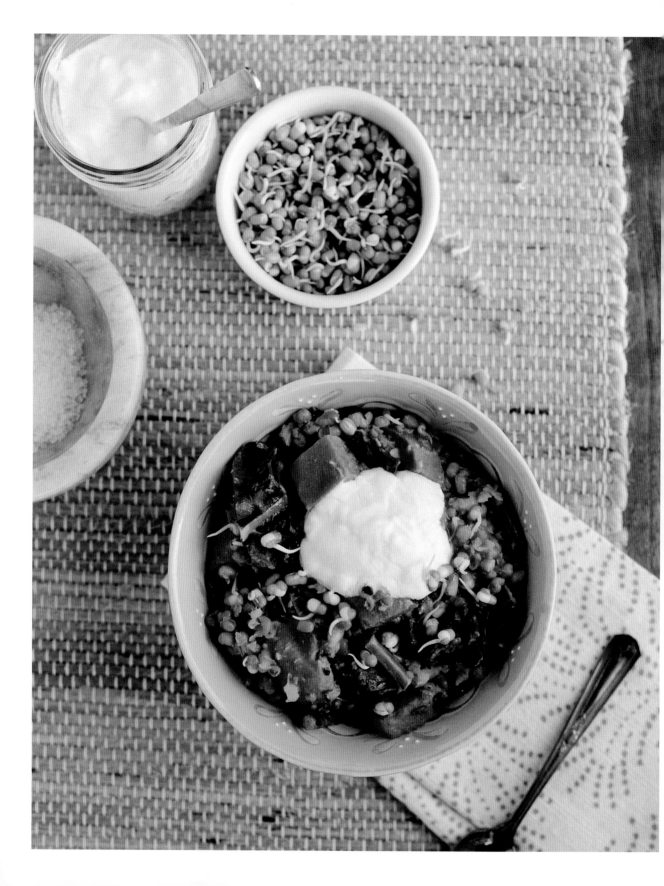

sprouted mung dal with yogurt

serves 4

Sprouted mung beans are easy to grow and lend a fresh, energizing atmosphere and a slight crunch to this rich winter stew. The energy of the sprout is light, mobile, and full of prana, life force. Deep in the winter, growing mung sprouts takes only a little effort and adds bright qualities to your diet.

5 cups water or broth

1 cup green mung beans, rinsed and soaked overnight

1 tsp Winter Spice Mix (see page 283)

2 cups cubed sweet potatoes, white potatoes, or carrots

4 leaves Swiss chard

1 tbsp ghee

½ tsp cumin seeds

½ tsp black mustard seeds

½ tsp salt

½ cup fresh Sprouted Mung Beans

4 tbsp yogurt for garnish

In a large saucepan on high heat, begin to boil the water or broth. Drain the soaked mung beans and add to the water or broth, along with the spice mix. Boil for 10 minutes. Add cubed potatoes or carrots. Turn heat to low, partially cover, and set the timer for 30 minutes. While the dal simmers, slice chard into thin ribbons and add for the remaining simmer time, partially covered.

In a small frying pan, warm the ghee on medium heat and sauté the cumin and mustard seeds until you can smell them, just 2-3 minutes. If the mustard seeds are popping out, cover the pan.

Pour the spiced ghee into the pot with the beans and vegetables. Add the salt and the sprouted beans, partially cover, and boil until the timer goes off.

Serve as a stew, perhaps over rice, with a tablespoon-sized dollop of yogurt on top of each serving.

fresh sprouted mung beans

Beans grew on a vine and were picked and dried. Now the bean is a seed, with dormant, potential energy until it gets soaked and watered. Sprouting awakens the energy of the seed and makes it a living food again.

Start with beans that aren't old and stale. Shop somewhere with good turnover in the bulk foods department. A place that is generally busy and has a large bulk section is likely to fit the bill. Old beans will refuse to sprout; they have lost their mojo.

Soak ½ cup of beans in 1 ½ cups water overnight. In the morning, drain and rinse the beans in a strainer or colander. Spread them out in a thin layer on the bottom of the colander or strainer, place a wide bowl underneath to catch drips, and a towel over the top. Leave out on the counter all day and night to sprout.

The next morning, rinse and drain the sprouts again. Cover with a towel and repeat the process. Within 48 hours or so (depending on how warm your kitchen is) the beans will begin to grow little white tails. It's best to eat the sprouts before the tails grow longer than ¼ inch. If you are not ready to eat them, you can refrigerate them in a glass storage container for a few days.

I generally make sprouts once or twice a week in winter. It's great to enjoy fresh produce from your own kitchen even in the depths of this season.

GET YOUR SPROUT ON

Sprouting has a rhythm, and once you are used to doing it, you won't forget to rinse the beans. Consider putting them in a bowl to soak when you get home for the day or before you go to bed. In the morning, rinse them and place them on top of the fridge (a nice warm place), covered with a towel. When you get home later that day, rinse them again. They should be sprouting by the following morning and ready for eating anytime that day, or you can let the tails grow another day or two, until you are ready to make Sprouted Mung Dal. Your sprouts will thank you for bringing them to such a beautiful finish.

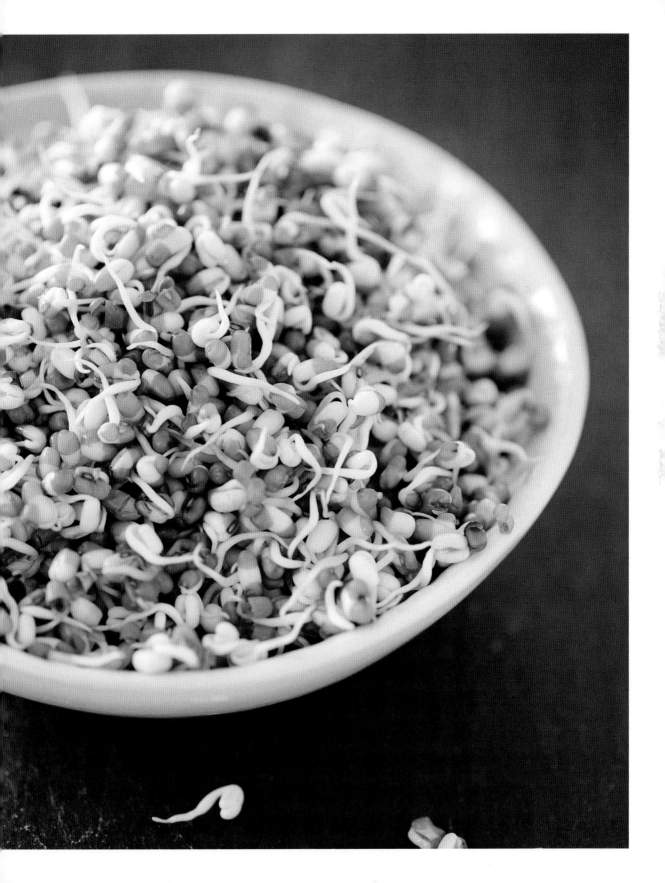

noodle bowl with toasted nori and mineral gomasio

serves 2

This recipe gets you working with the world of sea vegetables, high in minerals and B vitamins and a staple of a winter vegetarian diet. The taste of sea vegetables is sweet and salty, lending water to the body in dry times of year. The soup contains dried sea vegetables, and the two condiments, Toasted Nori and Mineral Gomasio, can be used to enrich any winter meal. Sea vegetables do not appear in the Ayurvedic texts, but those who live along the coast will do well to take advantage of this local food, rich in iodine, a key mineral for thyroid health.

SUPPER

NOODLE BOWL

4 cups water

8 oz tofu, cut into 2-inch triangles or ½-inch cubes

2 cups chopped vegetables: leafy greens cut into strips, carrots, daikon radishes

½ cup dried sea vegetables (sea palm and wakame both work well)

2 hearty handfuls of rice noodles, kelp noodles, or Zucchini Noodles (see page 186)

2 tbsp red miso

Bring the water to a boil in a large saucepan. Add the tofu, chopped vegetables, and sea vegetables. Reduce heat to medium and simmer, covered, about 10 minutes. Add noodles for the last 2 minutes of cooking and simmer until the noodles and the vegetables are al dente. Remove from heat.

In a small bowl, add just enough hot (not boiling) water to the miso to make a thin paste, about ¼ cup. Add this miso paste to the soup pot and stir. Boiling miso kills the enzymes, so it is important to add after taking the soup off the heat, just before serving.

Ladle into 2 large soup bowls and serve with Toasted Nori, if you like, and Mineral Gomasio.

SEASONAL RECIPES AND ROUTINES

TOASTED NORI

For this optional condiment, toast 2 sushi nori sheets by waving them over a stovetop burner until they turn bright green and crispy, just a few seconds. If you put the nori too close it will blacken—especially if you're using a gas burner. Toasted Nori can be used as a crispy side dish or crumbled on top of the soup before serving. I like to tear the sheets into quarters and pile on a small plate.

MINERAL GOMASIO

½ cup sesame seeds

1 tsp finely ground salt

1 tbsp dulse flakes

Dry roast the sesame seeds in a heavy-bottomed pan (cast iron works well) on medium-low heat, stirring constantly, until they begin to brown, just a few minutes. Cool completely, then halfway crush sesame seeds by hand with a mortar and pestle or by whizzing briefly in a spice-dedicated coffee grinder. Transfer to a small mixing bowl and stir in the salt and dulse flakes.

Store in a shaker jar at room temperature.

NOTE: Most health food stores carry dulse, nori, and wakame in the Japanese or Asian food department. See "Resources" (page 320) for culinary seaweed sources.

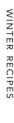

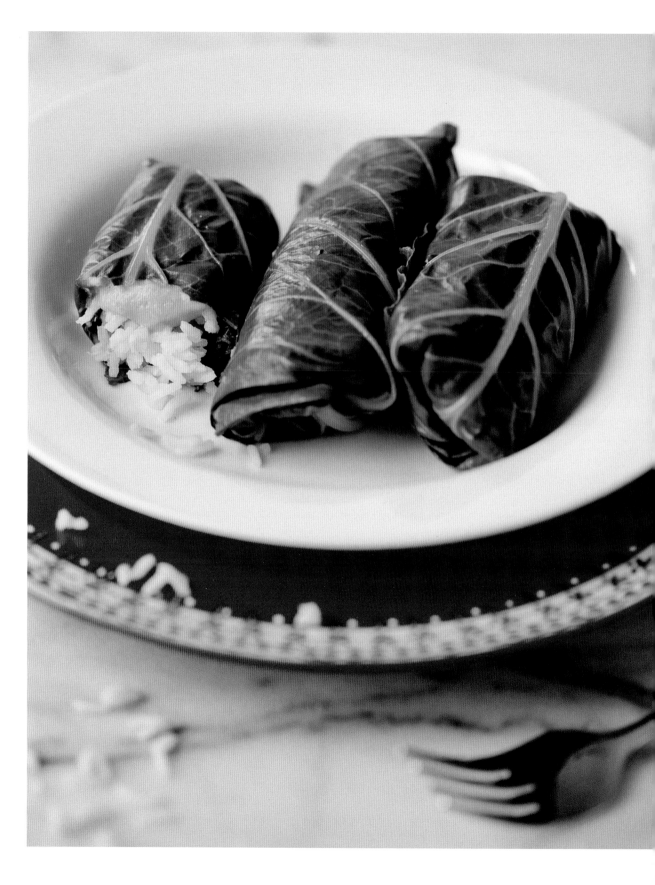

collard wraps with red lentil pâté

makes 4

Once you get the concept, you can make almost anything into a collard wrap, a cabbage wrap, or, in summer, a lettuce wrap. Red miso is very salty, sour, and slightly heating, and collards are one of those deep greens that is still in good shape in the winter, so this recipe makes a nourishing winter choice—but think of incorporating the collard wrap freely in all seasons. Wrapping kichari in collards is a quick way to change up a dal and rice routine.

RED LENTIL PÂTÉ

½ cup red lentils

¾ cup water

2½ tsp Winter Spice Mix (see page 283)

1 tbsp sesame tahini

juice of ½ small lemon

1½ tbsp red miso dissolved in 1 tbsp hot water

Rinse and soak lentils overnight. Drain and rinse. In a medium saucepan, bring the water to a boil. Add the lentils and spice mix. Simmer on low heat, covered, 30 minutes, until lentils are soft and water is absorbed. Remove from heat and cool a bit. Add the tahini, lemon juice, and miso paste and work in with a hand blender if you want your pâté creamy, with a fork if you want it with more texture. Add more water to the pâté if you prefer a thinner consistency.

COLLARD WRAPS

4 large collard leaves

1 cup cooked basmati rice

½ cup shredded carrots, cabbage, or beets (optional)

Bring 1 cup water to a boil in a large saucepan with a steaming basket inside.

Cut the stems off the collard leaves, and if you have delicate digestion, cut the thick part of the stem out of the middle too—a notch 1-2 inches up into the leaf will still let you use it for a wrap. Place the collard leaves inside the steaming basket and cover the pot. Steam on medium-low heat for 3 minutes. Take off the heat and remove leaves with tongs. The leaves should be bright green—do not overcook them.

TO MAKE THE WRAPS:

For each wrap, flatten a collard leaf and spread ¼ cup lentil pâté and ¼ cup rice up the middle in a rectangular shape. To add crunch, sprinkle on ⅛ cup shredded carrots, cabbage, or beets. Turn up the two short ends first, then roll up like a burrito, as shown in the photographs.

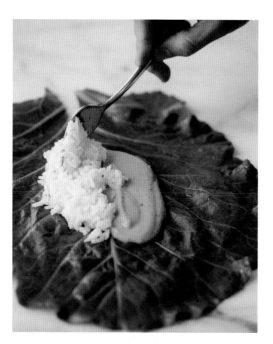
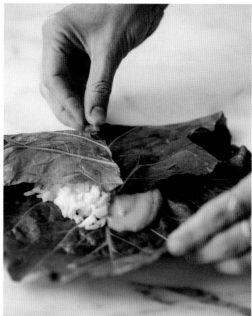
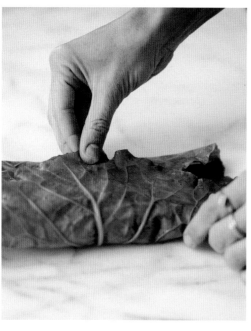
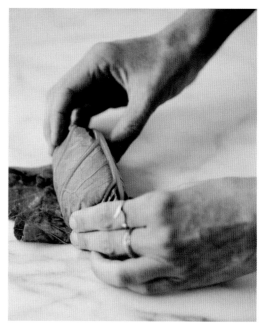

mixed potato pie with roasted maple almonds

serves 6

If your farm friends bring you lots of potatoes this winter, here is a deliciously sweet and savory way to serve up a bunch of potatoes for family and guests. White potato is light, cool, and dry and a member of the nightshade family. Nightshades are slightly poisonous when consumed in excess and promote inflammation, so they only appear in moderation in Ayurvedic cooking. This recipe integrates the beneficial sweet potato, which is not a nightshade. Always balance the dry, light, and cool qualities by serving potato dishes well oiled and with something of a sweet taste. The Roasted Maple Almonds not only look and taste wonderful but also balance the qualities of white potatoes.

ROASTED MAPLE ALMONDS

½ tsp Everyday Sweet Spice Mix (see page 118)

2 tbsp maple syrup

1 cup raw almonds

¼ tsp sea salt

1 tbsp coconut sugar or maple sugar

Preheat the oven to 350 degrees. Line a baking sheet with parchment paper. In a medium-size mixing bowl, mix together the Everyday Sweet Spice Mix and maple syrup. Add the almonds to the spiced maple and coat thoroughly. Mix together the salt and sugar and combine with the almonds. Spread the mixture on the lined baking sheet and roast for 10–12 minutes. Remove from oven and set aside. When cool, coarsely chop the almonds.

MIXED POTATO PIE

2 tbsp ghee, plus extra to grease the dish

2 cups cooked sweet potato, mashed (to roast your sweet potatoes, see The Yam Bomb, page 223)

2 tsp Winter Spice Mix (see page 283) or Everyday Sweet Spice Mix (see page 118)

1 egg (optional)

sea salt and ground black pepper to taste

1 medium white potato

Lightly grease the sides and bottom of a 9-inch pie dish with ghee. Using a food processor or hand masher, combine the mashed sweet potatoes, ghee, spice mix, egg, and salt and pepper and mix until well combined. With the skin on, slice the white potato into ⅛-inch thick slices. Layer the white potato slices on the bottom of the pie dish, overlapping the slices so the bottom of the dish is fully covered. Carefully spoon the mashed sweet potato mixture on top of the white potato slices, spread evenly to the sides of the pie dish, and smooth the top.

Bake on the top rack at 350 degrees for 40 minutes, or until the top begins to brown. Remove it from the oven, top with the coarsely chopped Roasted Maple Almonds, and allow to cool slightly before slicing.

Set out the remaining almonds in a bowl for those who would like to add more.

sweet potato bisque

serves 2

If you feel cold and hungry, this soup will comfort you—it's like having dessert as a meal. Sweet taste is the building block of a cold weather diet, balancing dry, hard, rough qualities. The heavy, oily hit from a bit of cream served warm and spiced here will nourish the deep tissues. Kids like it, too.

2 cups vegetable broth

½-inch piece fresh gingerroot, peeled and roughly chopped

¼ cup heavy cow's cream or coconut milk

1 medium-size or 2 small baked sweet potatoes (2 cups), skin optional

½ tsp turmeric

dash of nutmeg

dash of salt and pepper (optional)

2 tsp ghee

extra cream or coconut milk for garnish

Warm the broth, chopped gingerroot, and cream or coconut milk in a medium-size saucepan on medium-high heat. Slice the baked sweet potatoes into 4–5 pieces each and add to the pot to warm. Add spices, salt and pepper, if using, and ghee and simmer until the liquid boils. Remove from heat and use a hand blender to process to a smooth consistency, making sure to puree the gingerroot well.

Serve in 2 soup bowls with a tiny extra drizzle of cream or coconut milk on top.

NOTE: If you include the sweet potato skin in the soup, the color won't be as pleasing—it will be more brown than orange. I like to pull the skins off the baked sweet potatoes and eat them hot, on the side with ghee, my own version of "potato skins."

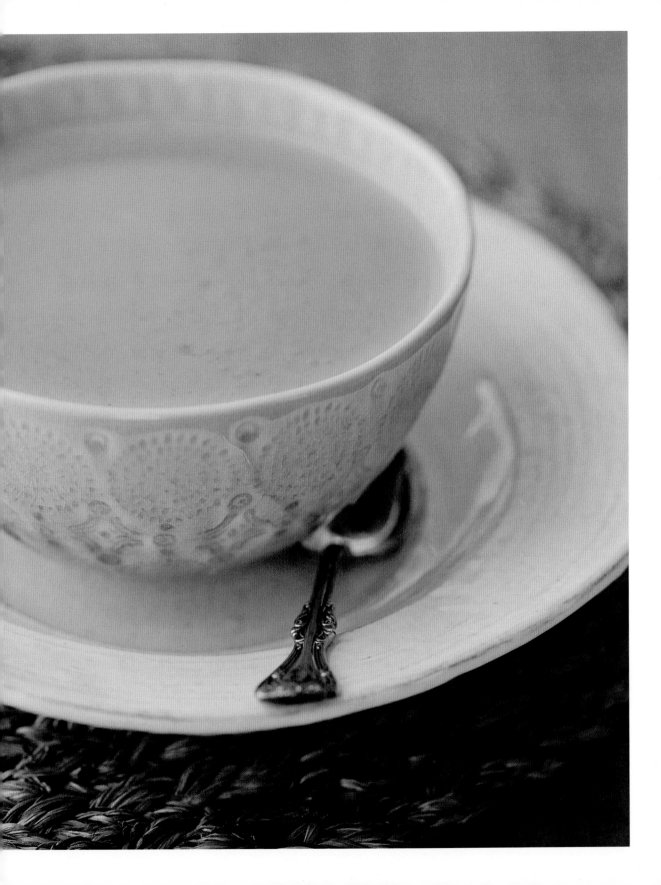

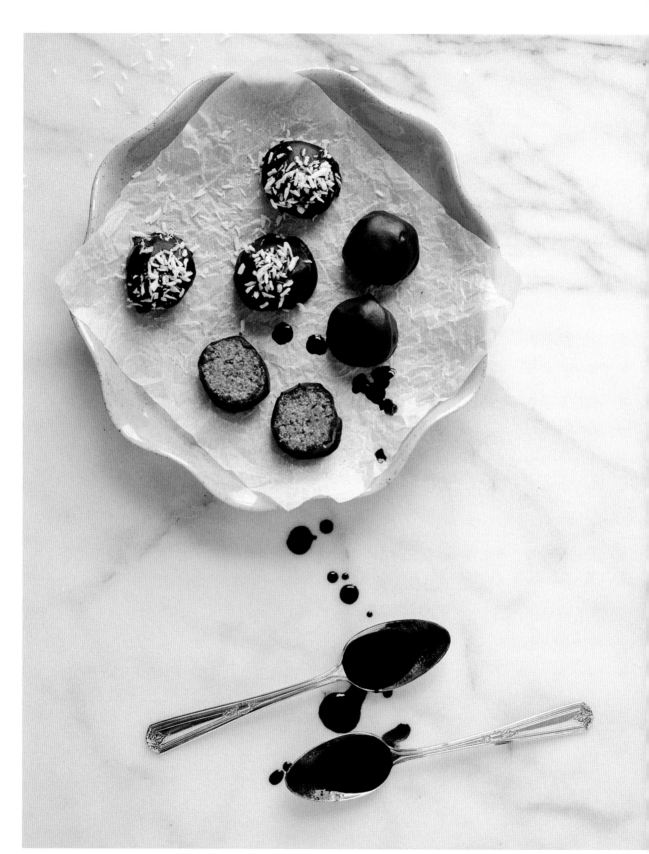

sunbutter truffles

makes about 12

Peanut butter often appears in treats, but the peanut, known as the "groundnut" in India, is not recommended in Ayurveda. The peanut is actually a legume; it is considered difficult to digest and increases heavy, dense, slow qualities. You will not miss peanut butter in this treat that calls for sunflower seeds and almonds instead. Sunbutter Truffles are so good, you may eat an extra one but not feel heavy because sunflower seed butter is lighter than any nut butter. The chocolate coating must stay refrigerated to keep from melting.

SUNBUTTER FILLING

- 2 tsp melted coconut oil
- ½ cup sunflower butter
- 1 tbsp raw honey
- 1 tsp pure vanilla extract
- ¾ cup almond meal
- ½ tsp cinnamon
- 2 tsp ashwagandha

CHOCOLATE COATING

- 3 tbsp melted coconut oil
- 1 tbsp + 2 tsp maple syrup
- 1 tbsp + 2 tsp cacao powder
- shredded coconut for decoration (optional)

Melt the coconut oil by standing the jar in hot water. In a small bowl, mix together 2 tsp melted coconut oil, sunflower butter, honey, and vanilla. Add the almond meal, sprinkle with cinnamon and ashwagandha, and stir to combine. Cover and place in the freezer for 45 minutes.

Cover a cookie sheet with a piece of parchment paper. Meanwhile, make the chocolate coating in a bowl by whisking with a fork the remaining 3 tbsp coconut oil with the maple syrup and cacao powder. Prepare it for dipping by placing the bowl inside a larger bowl of warm water. This will keep the coating from solidifying while you work. Take care not to get any water inside the chocolate.

With the chilled sunflower butter mixture, shape 1-inch balls and drop them, one at a time, into the chocolate. Using two spoons, roll the ball until it is totally coated, then lift it out and lay it on the papered cookie sheet. If desired, sprinkle coconut over the top before coating hardens.

Keep refrigerated until serving.

NOTE: These truffles contain ashwagandha, an adaptogenic herb known for its ability to nourish the deep tissues (bone, nervous tissue, reproductive tissue) and help the body cope with stress. Due to its warming energy, its use is especially indicated in fall and winter. If you don't have any, substitute 1 tsp almond meal for 2 tsp of the herb.

almond ginger macaroons

makes 12

With the addition of cacao nibs, these crunchy, chewy, flourless, sugarless macaroons leave nothing to be desired. Seriously! Fresh ginger adds a little kick and improves digestion. This is a great recipe to make for a holiday gathering, as they travel well in a storage container.

¾ cup almond meal

¼ cup unsweetened shredded coconut

¼ tsp baking powder

⅛ tsp salt

¼ cup dehydrated sugarcane or coconut sugar

2 tbsp cacao nibs

1 egg or 1 flax "egg" (see below)

1½ tbsp coconut oil

¼ tsp pure vanilla extract

1 tsp finely grated fresh gingerroot

Preheat the oven to 375 degrees. Lightly grease a cookie sheet with coconut oil.

In a small mixing bowl, combine the dry ingredients.

In a medium-size mixing bowl, beat the egg with a fork until fluffy.

Stir the oil, vanilla, and ginger into the egg. Pour the dry ingredients into the wet ingredients, stirring just until combined.

Use a large spoon to drop in tablespoon-size balls 2–3 inches apart on the cookie sheet. Press each ball down gently with a fork to flatten the bottom. Bake for 8–10 minutes, until cookies are lightly browned. Cool before removing from the sheet.

To make 1 flax "egg": In a blender carafe, combine 1 tbsp ground flaxseeds with 3 tbsp water and blend on high for 2 minutes.

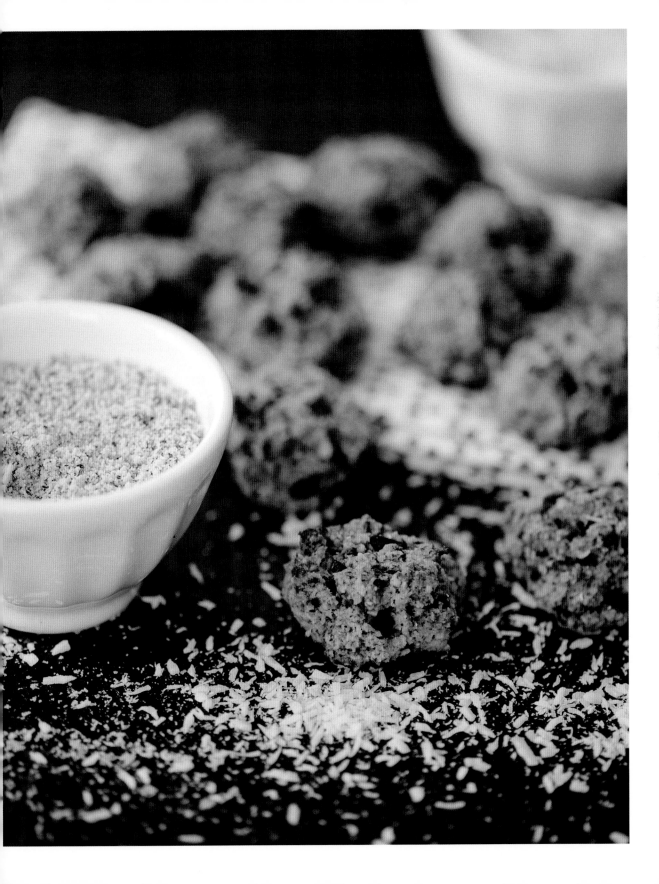

chocolate bark

The joys of melting chocolate chips and sprinkling different nuts and fruits over them to make bark at holiday time can never be underestimated. This love inspired me to create a recipe made with beneficial fat and unrefined sugar. May the spirit of the holidays live on without challenging your gut.

TREATS

½ cup coconut oil, melted

¼ cup maple syrup

¼ cup finely ground cacao powder

1 tsp cinnamon, cardamom, or ginger powder or 1 drop pure peppermint oil (optional)

dried cranberries, chopped nuts, hemp seeds, orange zest, candied ginger (note: candied ginger often contains white sugar), or dried lavender for decoration

Line a baking sheet with parchment or wax paper.

Whisk together the melted coconut oil, maple syrup, cacao powder, and spice powder or peppermint oil, if using, in a medium bowl. If your kitchen is chilly, you must move quickly so the chocolate doesn't begin to harden or else stand the bowl inside a larger bowl of hot water while you work.

Pour the chocolate mixture onto the paper-lined baking sheet and spread with a spatula to make a ¼-inch layer. Sprinkle your decorations on top. Refrigerate until hard, about 20 minutes. You should be able to touch the chocolate without leaving a fingerprint. Remove from the refrigerator and break into pieces with your hands—it works better than chopping.

Keep bark refrigerated so it doesn't melt.

NOTE: Coconut oil has been separated from the meat and fiber of the nut. Coconut butter is the meat of the coconut and its naturally occurring oil blended together. The body is likely to absorb the pure oil better; however, your bark will hold solid at temperatures below 76 degrees if you substitute coconut butter for the oil in this recipe. If you plan to take your bark out at a party or make it for gifts, it will be more stable at room temperature if made with coconut butter.

stuffed dates

serves 2

Sweet tooth got you? Need to whip up a quick dessert? These fancy dates are dense, moist, and deeply satisfying without containing any refined ingredients. Dates are known as an aphrodisiac in Ayurveda, and they increase rajas, or excitability of the mind. Best enjoyed in moderation, Stuffed Dates contain minerals, fats, and natural sweetness that bolster the system through the cold months.

....●●●●●..

4 Medjool dates

4 tsp raw almond butter

4 whole almonds or cashews

dash of Everyday Sweet Spice
    Mix (see page 118) or
    cinnamon

Cut a 1-inch slice lengthwise in each date and remove the pit. Stuff 1 tsp almond butter into each slit, letting it stick out the top a bit. Press an almond or cashew into the almond butter.

To serve, arrange the dates on a plate and sprinkle a dash of spice mix or cinammon over all.

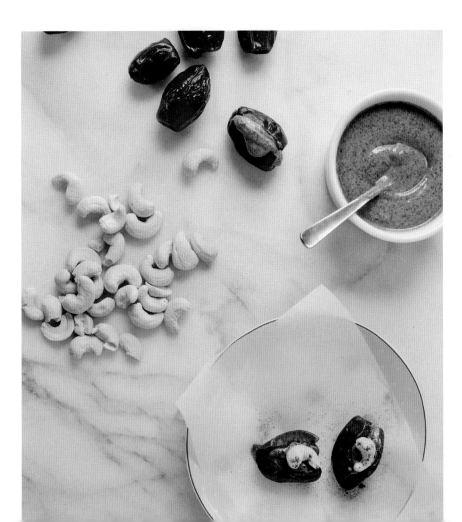

winter digestive tea

serves 2

This tea is a true winter warmer for the body. Cumin is known for its ability to help the body eliminate mucus–especially helpful in late winter, when mucus begins to accumulate.

2 cups water

½-inch piece fresh gingerroot

½ tsp cumin seeds

½ tsp fennel seeds

½ tsp cinnamon

Bring 2 cups of water to a boil in a small saucepan. Coarsely chop the gingerroot and add to the water; don't worry about removing the skin. Add the cumin seeds, fennel seeds, and cinnamon to the water. Reduce heat to low and simmer 10 minutes or longer if you prefer a strong flavor.

Strain hot tea into two mugs for serving. Take 6 ounces with or after meals.

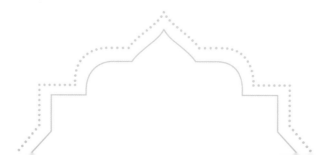

winter rejuvenating tonic

serves 2

Traditionally this tonic is taken in the evening, sometimes with the addition of building herbs, such as a teaspoon of ashwagandha, to support ojas, the nutrient "cream" of our bodies. If you are a smoothie maker, try this warm variety in place of cold, fruity versions, which freeze the gut and make you cold. Serve as a filling breakfast, a rich dessert, or a tempting snack for kids. Those who don't tolerate dairy products can substitute any nondairy milk.

· •●•●• ·

3–4 Medjool dates

10 almonds, soaked overnight

1 cup whole milk or Everyday Almond Milk (see page 114)

½ tsp Everyday Sweet Spice Mix (see page 118)

1 tsp ashwagandha (optional)

In a small bowl, soak the dates in warm water for 20 minutes. Remove the pits from the soaked dates.

Drain the almonds and remove the skins. They will slide right off between your fingers after soaking.

In a small saucepan, warm the dates, almonds, milk, spice mix, and ashwagandha, if using, on medium heat. When the milk is hot, remove from heat and blend with an immersion hand blender to smoothie consistency or process in a blender carafe until almonds and dates disappear.

Serve in a big mug. You've got a warm winter smoothie!

NOTE: Some find 1 cup of whole milk to be a bit too heavy or fatty for the digestive system. Rather than buy denatured, reduced fat milk, just dilute the whole milk with water to the consistency you prefer.

masala chai

serves 4

Some things should never be compromised. The perfect cup of chai offers a joie de vivre not to be tampered with. This recipe contains cow's milk, a healthy dose of sweetener, and black tea "dust," the Indian type of finely ground black tea leaves. Over the years, I have made many milk-free and caffeine-free variations: chai with rooibos, green tea, soy milk, almond milk—you name it. But I simply must offer you the real thing. You can omit the tea and still have a beneficial spiced milk, an excellent dessert. Do enjoy playing with this chai recipe, and soon you will make it your own with a unique choice of spices.

4 cups water

1 cup whole milk

1½ tbsp Indian-style fine tea dust or 3 tbsp loose leaf black tea (Brooke Bond Red Label is the choice of most Indian households)

2 tbsp coconut sugar

BASIC CHAI SPICES

½ tsp ginger powder or freshly grated ginger

½ tsp cinnamon

5 green cardamom pods, crushed

FANCIER ADDITIONS

2 whole cloves

½ tsp fennel seeds

dash of nutmeg (powdered or freshly ground)

My Secret Ingredient: 1 tsp coriander powder

In a medium-size saucepan, bring the water to a boil over high heat. Add all of the spices. Turn the heat down to low and simmer the spices for 10 minutes minimum. Turn the heat up to medium, add the milk, bring the liquid just to a boil again, and turn the heat down to low. Add the tea and sugar. Stir to dissolve. Do take care, because once you add the milk it can foam up suddenly. Do not leave it unattended until you are sure it's on a gentle simmer and not going to boil over. If I had a buck for every time I've blown up the chai pot... I'm trying to save you from the same fate. Simmer, uncovered, for 5–7 minutes. (The shorter time produces less caffeine and less drying astringency.) Take off the heat and pour through a fine strainer into another pot.

To serve, ladle into 4 small chai mugs from the new pot.

NOTE: I often bring 1 cup of water to boil the night before, add the spices, turn off the heat, and then let them steep overnight. In the morning, I add the milk, the rest of the water, and bring to a boil again.

ON MY SECRET INGREDIENT

Most self-respecting chai wallahs have a secret ingredient, and I am divulging mine. I picked this up from a yoga teacher in Rishikesh in 1998. He called his chai, with the addition of liver-boosting coriander powder, "yogi tea." I was sold and have made chai with this spice ever since.

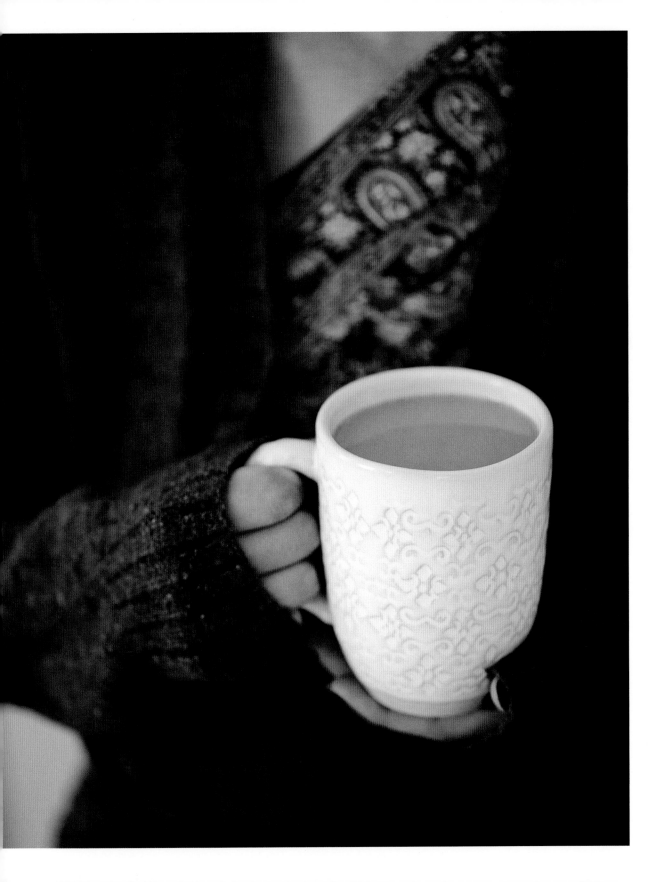

saffron lassi

serves 2

The flavor of a Saffron Lassi is subtle, yet exotic. The golden color is pleasing and invigorating. The stigmas, or fine threads of the saffron plant's flowers, are prized for their aphrodisiac and rejuvenating qualities—both of which we can use in the winter. I haven't called for saffron in many recipes, as it is expensive and not easy to find. But in this case, it's worth a try.

¼ cup organic whole milk yogurt
1 cup water, room temperature
1 pinch saffron threads
1 tsp maple syrup (optional)

In a 16-ounce wide-mouth mason jar, churn all the ingredients together for 1 minute with a hand blender, or use a carafe blender.

Pour into 2 glasses and serve at room temperature.

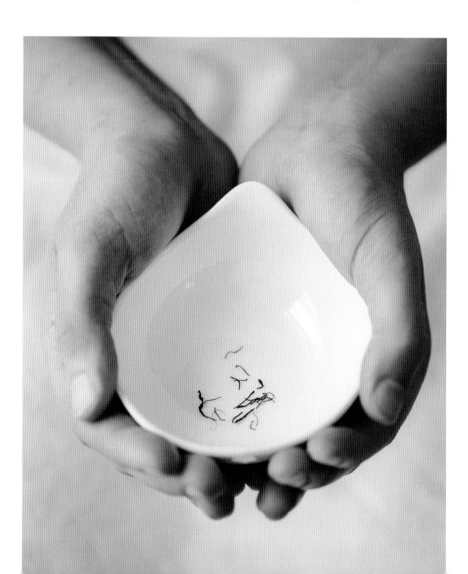

winter ayurvedic spice mix and salts

Welcome, winter spices! Salt, sweet, and sour are the tastes that ease the winter. Both of the blends here contain a hearty dose of salt and a bit of natural sweetness to go nicely with all your winter cooking. Winter is the time of year to be generous with spices.

WINTER SPICE MIX

makes ¼ cup

1 tbsp coriander seeds
1 tbsp cumin seeds
1 tbsp turmeric powder
½ tsp salt
½ tsp dehydrated sugarcane
1 tsp ginger powder
1 tsp black pepper (optional)

Dry roast the coriander and cumin seeds in a heavy-bottomed pan over medium heat until you can smell them, a few minutes. Cool completely. Combine with the other ingredients and grind to a uniform consistency in a spice-dedicated coffee grinder or by hand with a mortar and pestle.

Store in a small glass spice jar with a shaker top.

WINTER SALTS

makes ⅓ cup

2 tbsp dried rosemary
2 tbsp dried marjoram or oregano
1 tbsp sea salt
1 tbsp dehydrated sugarcane or maple sugar
1 tbsp black pepper

Mix the dried herbs, salt, sugar, and pepper together in a small glass shaker jar. Grind in a mortar and pestle first, if needed, to a uniform consistency. Many of the recipes in this section call for Winter Salts; however, you may also choose to keep the jar on the dining table as a condiment.

Keep a fresh pepper grinder on the table in winter and spring, filled with tricolored peppercorns. You can use it to grind 1 tablespoon for this recipe.

green mango ginger chutney

makes 16 ounces

Shopping for green mangoes always signals the beginning of a beautiful thing. Pick mangoes that are quite hard and have a fully green skin. When I am ready to make a big batch of this chutney for a winter's month, I plan it on a day when I can be home long enough to boil the cauldron for a while. A few hours of chutney preparation gives you a bounty of flavor that lasts for weeks in the refrigerator. I recommend making this chutney towards late winter, when sweet, sour, and spicy qualities are appropriate. Put on some tunes and lose yourself in the rhythm of dicing for a while.

EXTRAS

4 green mangoes

optional heat: 2 small green chilies or ¼ tsp cayenne pepper

4-inch piece fresh gingerroot

½ cup apple cider vinegar

¾ cup dehydrated sugarcane

optional neutral spices:
1 tsp cinnamon, cumin, and/or coriander powder

Peel and chop the green mangoes into 1-inch cubes, small enough to cook down easily.

Chop the chilies up very small, if using. Remove some of the seeds if you want a less spicy chutney, without compromising the flavor.

Peel and chop up the gingerroot into skinny, ½-inch sticks, so the fibers of the root are in small pieces.

In a large saucepan, combine all the ingredients together and simmer on low heat, uncovered, until the mixture reaches a jamlike consistency, an hour or so. All the ingredients could also be simmered in a slow cooker overnight.

Cool and transfer to a 16-ounce mason jar, keep refrigerated.

NOTE: I recommend adding the optional heat or, for those with a hot internal environment, the optional neutral spices—but not both. Although that could be tasty, it would mean there's a lot going on in one condiment.

SEASONAL RECIPES AND ROUTINES

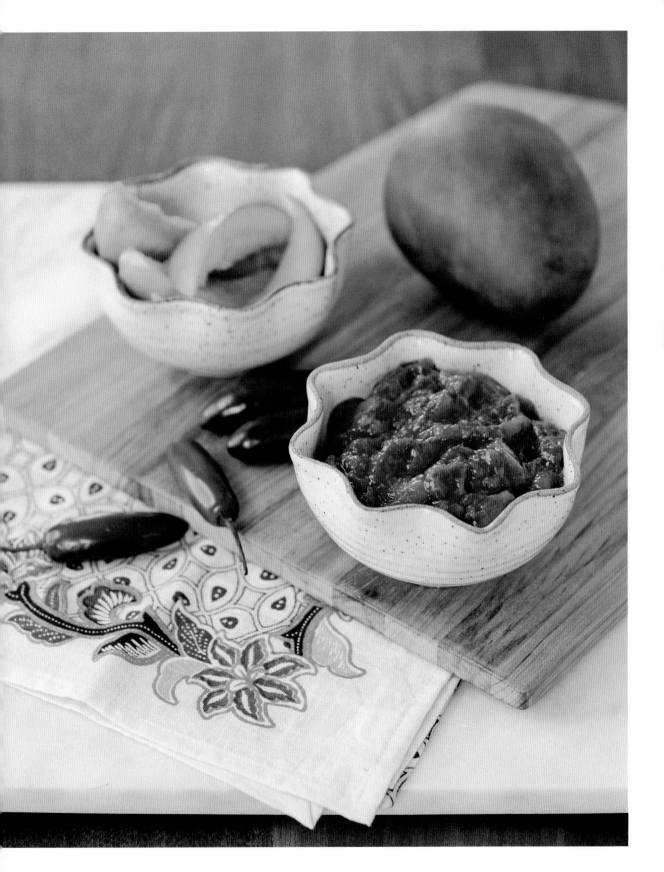

tomato date chutney

makes 16 ounces

This Punjab-inspired recipe is a great way to use home-canned tomatoes preserved from the summer garden. Fenugreek keeps the liver functioning well as the winter wears on. Try this chutney as an accent for dosa or alongside rice dishes. Tomato Date Chutney will keep for a week in the refrigerator.

1 tsp ghee
1 tsp fenugreek seeds
2 cups home-canned tomatoes
6 deglet noor dates, pitted
1 tsp salt
2 tsp fresh lemon juice

Melt the ghee in a medium-size frying pan or wide saucepan on medium heat. Toast the fenugreek seeds in the ghee, stirring constantly, until you can smell them, 2–3 minutes. Add tomatoes and salt to the ghee and stir to combine. Chop the dates into ¼-inch rounds and add to pan. Turn the heat down to low and simmer, uncovered, until the dates almost disappear, 15–20 minutes. Stir a few times while it simmers. When the chutney has reached a jamlike consistency, take off the heat and stir in the lemon juice.

Let it cool and transfer to a 16-ounce glass mason jar for storage—but try some hot with dosa before you put it away!

miso sesame dressing

makes 2-3 servings

Four of the six tastes are represented in this kingly condiment. Sesame's triple taste of sweet, bitter, and pungent, mixed with the sour of miso, creates a very balanced dressing, especially when served with the bitter, astringent tastes of dark leafy greens. Make this pairing a winter staple.

2 tsp sesame seeds

1 tbsp red miso dissolved in 1 tbsp hot water

¼ cup sesame oil (raw or refined for medium heat, not toasted)

¼ cup rice vinegar

½ tsp ginger powder

½ tsp cumin powder

dash of ume plum vinegar (optional)

In a small frying pan, toast the sesame seeds over medium-low heat, stirring constantly, until they begin to brown, just a few minutes.

Combine all the ingredients in a small bowl and whisk together with a fork or shake in an 8-ounce mason jar.

This dressing will keep for a week in the refrigerator. To serve, shake or stir vigorously before drizzling over an Everyday Steamed Salad Bowl, Red Lentil Pâté, sautéed greens, or cooked grains.

AYURVEDA AND FERMENTED FOODS

Fermented foods, such as miso and vinegar, increase heat in the body and balance stomach acid levels. Ferments are meant as a condiment only and can cause imbalance when taken in excess. Those whose digestive systems tend toward acidic might avoid fermented foods altogether or consume them as a strictly medicinal part of the diet in a 1 tbsp serving size.

In Ayurveda, fermented dairy products, such as buttermilk and homemade cheese, called "paneer," are a regular part of the diet. Pickled fruits and vegetables may be served in small quantities (1–2 tsp) to enliven the digestion in cold and rainy weather, while a few ounces of fresh buttermilk often appear at the end of midday meals (see Everyday Digestive Lassi, page 112).

In the Western diet, vinegar, wine, pickles, kombucha, aged cheeses, sauerkraut, and kimchi are often served in quantities that are less medicinal than they are habitual. Too much of a good thing—in this case, the sharp, penetrating qualities of fermentation—can cause a rise in the internal climate, which can promote imbalance in some cases.

Finally, remember that the longer something sits around, the more sour its taste. Traditional ferments are usually homemade and fresh, not store bought. Introduce fermented foods into the diet with moderation and find a local provider or learn how to make small batches at home.

Dinacharya Daily Practices

The following dinacharya, or daily practices, appear in the optimal order in which to do them. You do not have to practice them all; please consult the lifestyle guidelines in each seasonal chapter for more information on what times of year these procedures are most beneficial. Generally, tongue scraping and oiling of the skin are most important for everyday practice.

Tongue Scraper: A U-shaped, bevel-edged piece of copper or stainless steel used for cleaning the tongue.

Dry Brush: A stiff, natural bristle brush, with a wooden handle, used for exfoliating the skin.

Massage Oil: Be sure to buy organic, high-quality oil less than one year old for massage. Keep oils out of the sun. Visit the "Resources" section (page 320) for trusted mail order sources.

Neti Pot: Drugstores sell nasal irrigation kits with plastic pots and packets of salt (both handy for travel), but it's best to purchase a ceramic or stainless steel pot for home use. These can be purchased at most health food stores, or from a supplier in the Resources section of the book.

Glass Dropper Bottles: Sterile, empty glass dropper bottles can be purchased at some health food stores and herbal suppliers. Use to store sesame oil for the nose or rose hydrosol for the eyes.

Rose Hydrosol: A decoction made of the water of steamed rose petals, safe for use in the eyes and to flavor food. Hydrosol is different from rose water, which is made by adding rose essential oil to water and is unsafe for the eyes.

Tongue Scraping

Use a stainless steel or copper tongue scraper. First thing in the morning, before consuming any drinks, scrape the tongue five to six times, from as far back as you can get to the tip. Cover the entire surface of the tongue, especially way in the back. Press gently; do not disturb the tongue tissue. A mucus will likely appear on the scraper; rinse in the sink as needed.

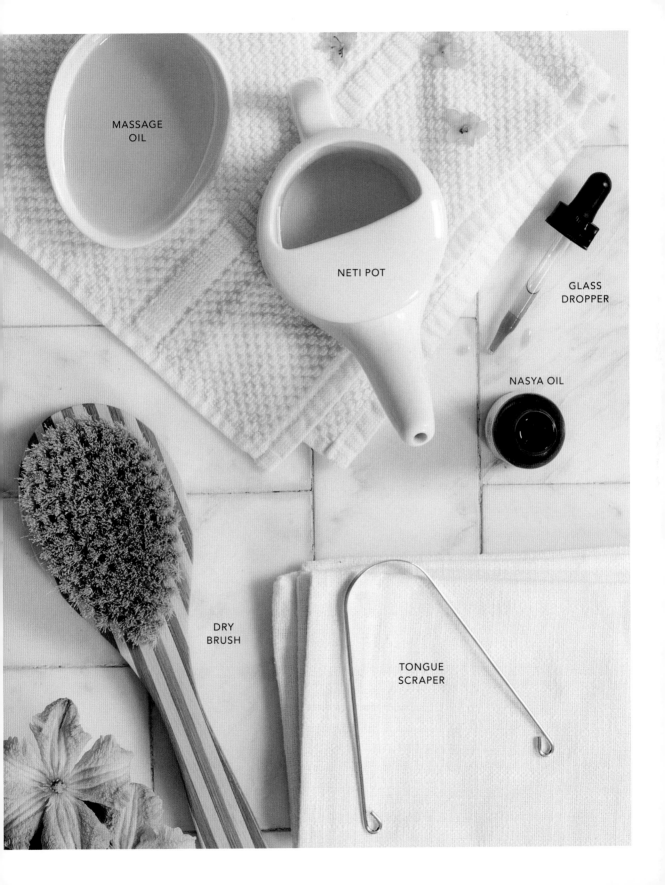

MASSAGE
OIL

NETI POT

GLASS
DROPPER

NASYA OIL

DRY
BRUSH

TONGUE
SCRAPER

After finishing, clean the scraper thoroughly with hot water and keep it near your toothbrush. Do not scrape the tongue at other times of day. Follow with tooth brushing and a cup of hot water or Easy Morning Beverage (page 110).

Wash the Eyes

Run cool water from the tap and rinse the eyes well by splashing the cool water over open eyes with your hands four or five times. Follow by blinking seven times and rolling the eyes in circles. Those with burning, itching, or redness of the eyes can spray or drop rose hydrosol into the eyes at this time. Be sure to purchase a hydrosol rather than water with rose essential oil added to it. Essential oils are not safe for the eyes.

Neti (Nasal Irrigation)

Think of neti, irrigation of the nasal passage, as being like flossing for your nose. Using a neti pot involves pouring a small amount of salt water from a ceramic or stainless steel pot through each nostril, dislodging accumulating mucus and impurities. I like to practice neti in the shower, when the warmth of the shower opens the nasal passage and any drips will be washed away.

Potential bugs can't get a hold on you when you use the neti pot. Practice neti in the morning, at the change of seasons, when the cold and flu season begins, and as needed through the spring and fall. Mucus-prone or allergic types will find they benefit from daily use of the neti pot, while dry types will need this only occasionally and will benefit more from nasya (see next page). This practice can also be used for a few days when immunity feels compromised. Not everyone needs it every day.

To practice, boil purified water and add enough cold purified water to be sure it is not too hot. You should be able to hold your finger in it without it feeling too hot. Be sure to check. Dissolve fine grain, pure sea salt completely in the warm water (neti pots come in different sizes, please read the instructions on yours to find the correct amount of salt). In the shower or at the sink, lean forward, keeping the back of the neck extended, so your whole torso is bending. Tip your head and place the spout into the top nostril and wait for the water to run out the other nostril.

If water is not draining easily after a few tries, refrain from practicing until you can get formal guidance. Let the water run out naturally. *Do not* forcibly blow the nose, as this can send the water in further. You may cover one nostril and simply exhale to help the last bit of water out. Tip the head the other way and repeat for the other nostril.

NOTE: Too much salt burns; too little leaves you feeling like you have swimmer's ear. Do not practice neti more than once a day.

Nasya (Oiling of the Nose)

Unless you experience congestion, always follow neti with nasya, applying sesame oil to the nostrils by swirling it in with a Q-tip or pinky fingertip and inhaling deeply. This will balance the drying effect of salt. Order oil from a supplier on the resource list (see page 320), or you can make your own nasya oil by decanting refined sesame oil into a sterile dropper bottle. Drop the oil onto your pinky, Q-tip, or directly into your nostril and do not touch the dropper. Even if you don't practice neti, take care to oil the nose while doing daily oil massage. Don't forget to bring your nasya oil on plane rides and to use before riding public transportation. The oil is generally good for one year.

Nasya is not indicated in cases of chronic congestion; better to see an Ayurvedic practitioner to help you discover the cause. But do take note that food allergies can cause congestion, and a seasonal cleanse might clear you up, as well as giving you an opportunity to discover what is causing the problem as you reintroduce certain foods to your diet after the cleanse.

Dry Brushing

This procedure is especially indicated in late winter and spring or in conditions of weight gain or water retention. Use a natural bristle dry brush (available in drugstores and health food stores) on dry skin. Beginning at the ankles and moving up toward the heart, make small, brisk circles to exfoliate and stimulate the skin of the entire body, especially the armpits and chest, inner thighs and groin, and anywhere stubborn fat tissue likes to hang around. Take three to five minutes and be firm, but do not disturb the skin. A rosy color should result. Practice anywhere from daily to once a week, before having your shower and oil massage.

Abhyanga (Oiling of the Skin)

If you do only one dinacharya practice, do this one. You will notice the oiling of the skin creates a protective, strengthening force field around you for the day.

It's best to apply warm oil thickly right before you shower or in the shower. The warm water will open the pores, and the massage will penetrate more deeply. Warm the oil by sitting a small container of it in a sink of hot water while you get undressed. Apply oil for 5 minutes before you shower, using long strokes along the bones and circular strokes on the joints. In cold weather, you might choose to keep a small plastic container of massage oil in your shower. When you're ready to perform your abhyanga, put the container on the shower floor and turn on the water, so you and the oil warm up together in the shower for a minute. Turn off the water; apply a palmful of oil to the entire body, including the ears and nostrils—but you may skip the rest of the face. Rub it in well for a few minutes, then turn on the warm water again, stand under it, and rub some more. Do not soap off your skin—just soap the hairy parts to remove the oil. Towel dry—lingering in your towel for a few minutes to let the skin absorb the oil, if necessary—get dressed, and go about your day.

WHAT KIND OF OIL TO USE

You may enjoy changing your massage oil with the seasons as indicated in the seasonal lifestyle guides, but here are a few general choices. Please be sure to do a patch test with any oil before applying to the entire body, to be sure you are not allergic.

Sesame oil: Traditionally sesame oil is favored for its ability to build strength and softness in the body. Sesame oil is warming and indicated for those who run cold and experience dry skin.

Sunflower and almond oil: These two lighter oils are neither heating nor cooling and are indicated for those who do not experience very dry skin.

Coconut oil: Coconut oil is cooling and indicated for those who run hot or have sensitive skin.

Special Abhyanga during a Seasonal Cleanse

The following practice, known as *snehana*, is recommended daily throughout a seasonal cleanse to quiet the nerves and to soften impurities and the channels that carry them out of the body, so they can be released.

Sneha means "love" in Sanskrit, and this ancient practice is literally an application of love. Taking the time for this kind of massage once a week throughout the year will greatly enhance the immune system, strengthen the nervous system, and help with pain management.

Warm ¼–½ cup organic sesame oil in a jar or bottle placed in hot water. Make sure the room you oil in is cozy and warm. Prepare the room and remove your clothes before you begin, to minimize the need to move (and the possibility of slicking surfaces with oil). Lay an old bath towel on the floor and sit down. Breathe deeply a few times and give thanks for the time and space to care for yourself in this way. Apply the warm oil to your body with love and patience. Rub it in well, especially in areas that trouble you. Beginning with the feet, work your way up the body, using long strokes along the bones, circular strokes on the joints, and wide clockwise circles on the chest and abdomen. Massage the face and head last, rubbing the oil into the scalp. Use your little fingers to put oil in the ears and nose. Half a cup will seem like a lot. Keep going until you don't think your skin can absorb anymore; this process may take 15 minutes. When you've massaged in all the oil, lie back on your towel and relax for 5 to 30 minutes. It takes at least 20 minutes for the body to absorb the oil, so after 15 minutes of massage, relax for at least 5 minutes. Burn a candle or play soft music. Now enjoy a hot shower, but wipe your feet first so you don't slip. Do not use soap; the hot water will remove any excess oil. Apply shampoo to hair before wetting to cut the oil. After you shower, pat yourself dry. Your skin may still seem a bit oily; massage the oil in further, and it will gradually be absorbed. Afterward, clean your bathtub or shower stall of residual oil to make sure no one slips!

NOTE: When your towel becomes very oily, it can create a fire hazard if you put it in the dryer after washing. Better you hang your abhyanga towels to dry and replace them periodically instead.

Seasonal Cleansing

These guidelines are applicable to both spring and fall cleansing.

FINDING THE TIME

Look at your calendar and find a week when you don't have any big events, deadlines, or air travel scheduled. You may need to cancel a social engagement or two, especially in the evening, to ensure you get enough rest. Staying up too late will make you hungry, tire you out, and reduce the efficacy of your cleansing period. If an engagement is unavoidable, bring the food you prepared along with you or order steamed vegetables, plain rice, hot water with fresh lemon, and clear soups at restaurants. During this time you have set aside, please don't feel shy about pulling out your own food at a shared meal. This is your opportunity for self-care, and you are not being rude or inconveniencing anyone by making specific choices about what you eat for a set period of time. You are inspiring!

It is generally difficult to identify a week with "nothing" going on, but still it's better to try to create a few days of space than to get discouraged by the calendar and better to bring your own food than to let shared meals and planned events overshadow your seasonal self-care.

DECIDING HOW LONG

Block off three to seven days for your cleanse, and take it one day at a time. If you have little body fat, experience extreme headaches, find yourself light-headed, or develop difficulty concentrating, you may need to stop your cleanse at three days. A cleanse is not a contest but an act of compassionate self-care, and even a day or two has a positive effect. Getting started is usually the hardest part, and being open to doing it for just a few days, rather than pushing yourself to the extreme, will ensure success.

TIPS FOR A SMOOTH CLEANSE

- Prepare a batch of Everyday Kichari in the morning. This one pot will become your three meals for the day. Eat a portion for breakfast, pack what you need for lunch, leave the rest in the pot for dinner (only store it in the refrigerator if you live in a hot climate).
- A vigorous oil massage in the morning wakes you up, while a gentle massage in the evening can help you sleep. Carve out 30 minutes each

day of your cleanse, at either time of day, to practice abhyanga. See Seasonal Self-Care 1, "Special Abhyanga during a Seasonal Cleanse" (page 292).

- Prepare and bring enough kichari to work. Lighter individuals or those with low blood sugar may need to eat four meals a day. *Especially* when you are new to cleansing, always pack an extra meal, to avoid finding yourself without enough food.
- Remember: rest and relaxation are key elements of detoxification. The body will not get rid of toxins until you carve out some time and create a restful, safe environment for detoxifying. If the physical body or nervous system is overworked, the body will continue to crave building, grounding qualities from heavier comfort foods, such as cheese, meat, and bread, to keep up with the pace you are setting.
- If you suffer from chronic congestion, note that food allergies can cause congestion, and a seasonal cleanse might clear that up, as well as give you an opportunity to see what is causing the problem as you reintroduce certain foods to your diet after the cleanse. If the congestion persists, see an Ayurvedic practitioner.

SPOTLIGHT ON *PANCHAKARMA*

Panchakarma means "five actions." It refers to the five actions traditionally used to remove excess dosha that has accumulated in the body: vomiting, purgation, cleansing of the nasal passage, and two types of enemas, cleansing and nutritive. Consult an Ayurvedic practitioner or find a panchakarma center to learn more (see "Resources," page 320), and do not undergo these actions without professional guidance.

Purvakarma is more appropriate for the do-it-yourself crowd (including most readers of this book). *Purva* means "before," and *purvakarma* refers to preparatory actions taken before panchakarma. These include eating a monodiet of kichari and practicing therapies such as abhyanga (oil massage) and *svedana* (sweating, which can be accomplished in a steam room or bath) to prepare the body for a forcible removal of aggravated dosha. Purvakarma assists the body in its natural process of alleviating accumulated dosha in three ways:

- It removes difficult-to-digest foods from the diet.
- It enables the body and its sense organs to relax and rest.
- It softens impurities and the channels that eliminate them.

For the seasonal cleanse set aside time at the change of seasons to give yourself oil massage, prepare simple, seasonal foods, and indulge in rest and quiet time. The spring and fall chapters guide you through how to gain the most benefit from these ancient practices.

Simple Spring Cleanse

As temperatures become consistently warmer, accumulated heavy/dense and sticky/moist qualities, which protected us from winter's cold, begin to soften. Your body prepares to break down and discharge what it no longer needs. The Simple Spring Cleanse maximizes your body's natural inclination to get rid of excess fat and mucus in spring. This is a three- to seven-day program of eating a monodiet of Everyday Kichari (see page 100), which has detoxifying qualities, and practicing daily dry brushing and oil massage. Dry brushing and oil massage will loosen impurities and stimulate your lymphatic system, the main line for detoxification. Spring cleansing is a preventive measure to ensure good health for the coming season.

You may find you need less food in the springtime and feel the desire to exercise a bit more during or soon after your cleanse. Listen to your body's natural cravings. If you had a long indulgent or sedentary winter, you will need to shed some heavy qualities by choosing bitter and astringent vegetables and getting your body moving.

TO PREPARE

Begin practicing the spring dinacharya, grind your Spring Spice Mix, and familiarize yourself with the spring shopping list. If you haven't made Everyday Kichari before, make a practice batch to get the hang of it.

If you feel you need more guidance during your cleanse or have questions about whether an Ayurvedic spring cleanse is for you, consult an Ayurvedic practitioner (see "Resources" on page 320).

THE DAILY MENU

- Have Easy Morning Beverage to start the day; no caffeine.
- Stick to a monodiet of Everyday Kichari, made with one spring vegetable per batch, and Spring Spice Mix (see page 158).
- Eat three meals each day. Lighter individuals or those with inconsistent blood sugar may need four daily meals—but no snacking in between. Do not eat if you are not hungry.
- Drink 6 ounces of hot Spring Digestive Tea with meals and/or sip from a thermos throughout the day.
- Sip warm water and ginger tea throughout the day—nothing cold.
- If you need more nourishment, have Everyday Cleansing Green Soup (page 108) or a Cleansing Green Juice (page 157) to augment the midday meal. Need variety? Try Barley Kanjee (page 89) for breakfast.

DAILY OIL MASSAGE

Set aside 30 minutes each day, all to yourself, to do your oil massage. See Seasonal Self-Care 1, "Dinacharya Daily Practices" (page 288), for complete instructions on how to practice abhyanga. If sesame oil is too heavy for use in spring or you feel lethargic after oiling, use a lighter oil, such as sunflower or grapeseed.

SPRING CLEANSE LIFESTYLE AND EXERCISE GUIDELINES

Avoid:
- Cold food and drink
- Extra salt. Use only the amount specified in the Ayurvedic recipes.
- Vigorous exercise. If you are very fit, do 50 percent of what you are used to.
- Eating between meals
- Eating too much at one time

Enjoy:
- Dry brushing the skin
- A sauna, steam room, or Epsom salts bath
- Walking or practicing gentle yoga
- Giving yourself a daily oil massage. This is important to help your body release impurities and calm your nervous system.
- Going to bed early, lying down an hour or two earlier than you are used to

Signs of a Successful Spring Cleanse:
- Any white coating on your tongue clears up.
- Your breath is fresh.
- You have regular bowel movements without gas or bloating.
- The whites of your eyes are clear.
- You feel brighter, more energetic.
- Any lingering sinus or chest congestion is gone.

When to Plan Your Spring Cleanse

If you live in a cold climate, make sure you wait until temperatures are consistently above freezing so your body won't have to restock its dense and sticky stores. In most areas, this can be as early as March or April, and in cooler climates, as late as May.

Short and Sweet Fall Cleanse

As temperatures cool, the body prepares to release excess fire and water elements that accumulated during hot, humid weather. The dry winds of fall can stir up the fire element and cause compromised immunity, inflammation, acidic digestion, skin problems, allergies, and a short temper. Assist your body in its natural release of hot, sharp, oily qualities with an Ayurvedic fall cleanse, which will also prepare you for the dry, cool, rough qualities of autumn. A fall cleanse bolsters the immune system during cold and flu season. It also improves digestion.

The fall cleanse is a three- to seven-day program of an Ayurvedic monodiet of kichari, daily oil massage, and plenty of rest and relaxation. As described earlier (page 100), kichari is a special food that both detoxifies and nourishes, allowing your system to recalibrate without any aggravation. Daily oil massage will loosen impurities and stimulate your lymphatic system, the main line for detox. Rest and relaxation are essential during the fall cleanse to allow your body's energy to feed the deep tissue layers, protecting your bones, nervous system, and reproductive organs.

Be sure to review Seasonal Self-Care 1 (page 308) before beginning your cleanse.

TO PREPARE

Begin practicing the fall dinacharya, grind your Fall Spice Mix, and buy a few vegetables from the fall shopping list. If you haven't made Everyday Kichari before, make a practice batch to get the hang of it.

If you need more guidance about whether an Ayurvedic fall cleanse is for you, consult an Ayurvedic practitioner (see "Resources" on page 320).

THE DAILY MENU

- Drink Easy Morning Beverage to start the day; no caffeine.
- Eat a monodiet of Everyday Kichari, made with one fall vegetable per batch, and Fall Spice Mix (see page 240).
- Eat three sit-down meals each day. Lighter individuals or those with inconsistent blood sugar may need four daily meals—but no snacking in between. Do not eat if you are not hungry.
- Drink 6 ounces of hot Fall Digestive Tea with meals and/or sip from a thermos throughout the day.
- Sip warm water and herbal tea throughout the day—nothing cold.
- If you need more nourishment, have Everyday Cleansing Green Soup or an Everyday Digestive Lassi to augment the midday meal. If you need variety, try plain Everyday Creamed Grain Cereal for breakfast.

DAILY OIL MASSAGE

Set aside 30 minutes each day to massage your body with oil and to oil your nose.
See Seasonal Self-Care 1 for instructions on abhyanga and nasya. Using plain
sesame oil in the nose will balance the dry qualities of the season and protect
from cold and flu bugs that like to cling to the inside of your nasal passages.

FALL CLEANSE LIFESTYLE AND EXERCISE GUIDELINES

Avoid:
- Cold foods and drinks
- Raw foods
- Spicy ingredients, such as hot sauce, chilies, and cayenne pepper
- Nightshades: tomatoes, bell peppers, eggplant, and white potatoes
- Vigorous exercise. For example, if you usually run, walk instead.
- Eating between meals
- Eating too much at one time

Enjoy:
- A nap if you need it
- A sauna, steam room, or Epsom salts bath
- Restorative yoga
- Sipping hot water
- Giving yourself a daily oil massage to release impurities and calm your
  nervous system
- Going to bed early, lying down an hour or two earlier than you are
  accustomed to

Signs of a successful Fall Cleanse:
- Any white coating on your tongue clears up.
- Your breath is fresh.
- You have regular bowel movements without gas or bloating.
- The whites of your eyes are clear and bright.
- You feel consistent energy levels, grounded and calm.
- Skin rashes and pimples clear up.

When to Plan Your Fall Cleanse

Late September and October are the best time, when the weather is consistently cool—but before temperatures reach freezing. Ayurveda does not
advise performing a cleanse when it is very cold out.

Tools and Techniques
for Everyday Ayurveda

Carafe Blender: A blender with a glass carafe has more power than a hand blender and is called for in recipes in which the ingredients are too hard or fibrous for a hand blender, such as juices and chutneys.

Food Processor: This tool takes up a lot of space, but it has the most power for grinding nuts and makes chunkier chutneys and smoother, thicker pâtés and hummus than a carafe blender.

Hand Blender: Also known as an immersion blender or stick blender (see equipment photo). Used to blend nut milks and to puree soups, a hand blender is quicker to clean than a carafe blender. Works especially well for hot soups, which can make a carafe too hot.

Pressure Cooker: A staple in an Indian kitchen, a pressure cooker cuts cooking time in half for legumes and hard vegetables, without requiring soaking, and ensures a well-cooked, easily digested bean.

Rice Cooker: An electric rice cooker can be preset to make rice or kichari by a certain time. This tool is a great time saver.

Graters and Grinders

Grater: Metal box graters are common, but a plane grater takes up less space in the kitchen. A good grater should have small and large grating options and be sturdy. Microplane graters work great for grating gingerroot.

Mortar and Pestle: Stone grinding is traditional in much of India's cooking, and it is still common to see home cooks sitting outside, grinding the day's ingredients. Everyday Ayurveda recommends that you enjoy the aromatic task of freshly grinding spices for your meals. A stone mortar and pestle will not retain scents, like wood does.

Spice Grinder: A coffee grinder reserved for spices, seeds, and nuts allows you to make large amounts of spice mixes quickly for storage.

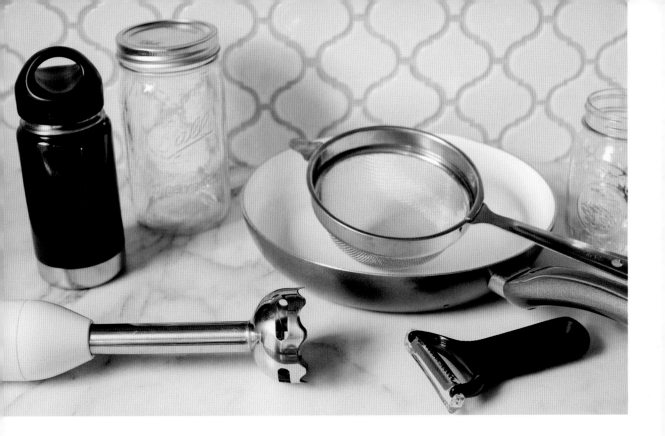

Pepper Mill: Freshly ground pepper at the table is a joy of life. Look for a wooden pepper mill and fill it with high-quality black or multicolor peppercorns.

Pots, Pans, and More

Saucepan: A soup pot with high walls, usually in two-, four-, and six-quart sizes. A four-quart pot is best for recipes that serve four or more, while a two-quart pan can be used to make smaller amounts. Favor high-quality stainless steel saucepans such as All-Clad brand and do not buy aluminum, which is soft, porous, and reactive to certain foods, which can create questionable chemical compounds in your food. It is worth the investment to buy a few good saucepans.

Frying Pan: A frying pan is broad and wide, with a short lip, and is used for steam sautéing and frying. "Green" frying pans with a ceramic nonstick covering are preferable to other nonstick surfaces. Get rid of your Teflon, which can create harmful chemical compounds if the coating breaks down into your food.

Cast Iron Frying Pan: Cast-iron pans have been favorable cooking tools for slow cooking, frying, and baking because of their resiliency and ability to distribute heat evenly. A well-seasoned pan will have a nonstick quality. My recipes call for a large size, which can be anywhere from fifteen to seventeen inches in diameter. A smaller diameter can be used, though you may need to increase cooking times.

Glass Baking Dish: My recipes call for an eight- by eight-inch square dish, as well as a nine-inch pie dish. One dish can substitute for the other in the recipes.

Fine Mesh Sieve: A colander's holes are too big for some grains and legumes, so a metal sieve or strainer is essential for rinsing these as well as vegetables.

Baking Sheet: Used for cookies; look for high-grade stainless steel, not aluminum. Some recipes call for lining with parchment paper.

Parchment Paper: Parchment paper is used for lining a cookie sheet to keep foods from sticking; it is preferable to wax paper for baking.

Muffin Tins: Generally available with six or twelve cups; most of my recipes make six muffins. Look for steel tins, not aluminum.

Muffin Cups: Some of my muffin batters are too dense to sit alone in a muffin tin and require lining with paper cups, which can be found in the baking aisle of the grocery store.

Kitchen Techniques

Almond Soaking: To soak almonds eight hours or overnight in cool water. Soaking releases enzymes in the nut and makes them easier to digest, not to mention delicious and versatile.

Destem: To remove the stems from large leafy greens. Hold the stem in one hand and cup the other hand around the bottom of the leaf. Gently squeeze and strip the leaf off the stem with one pull. Chop the leaf for cooking and discard the stem or save for broth.

Dry Roast: To roast spices lightly in a dry pan, just until they begin to release their oils and aromas.

Grind: To slowly break down spices, seeds, and nuts by hand in a mortar and pestle or in an electric grinder (use a coffee grinder that is reserved for spices or a small attachment for your food processor). Most spices in traditional Ayurvedic cookery are freshly ground by hand for each meal.

Hand Blend: To make a puree (or to churn yogurt with water) by immersing a hand blender in the cooking pot and processing food until smooth. Keep the blender submerged and turn it off before taking it out of the liquid. A tall canning wide-mouth jar works great for beverages.

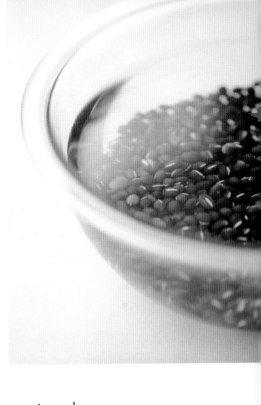

Quick Soak: To bring water and a grain or legume to a rolling boil for five minutes, then covering and letting sit for one hour. This will have the same effect as soaking overnight.

Rinse: To remove impurities from grains and legumes by rinsing with cool water. Add the dry item to a saucepan and cover with water. Agitate the water with your fingers until it becomes cloudy. Pour the water and grain or legume through a mesh strainer. Rinse under the faucet until the water runs clear.

Soak: To cut down cooking times by soaking grains and legumes in cool water anywhere from one hour (for grains and small beans) to overnight. Rinse the grains or beans well first, put them in a bowl with twice the amount of water, and cover. The longer an item soaks, the faster it will cook. Remember to reduce cooking water in the recipe if you soaked first. Any soak water that remains can be used for cooking.

Sprout: To soak dried foods such as nuts, seeds, and beans in fresh water to revive them, then rinsing daily until they grow tails. Sprouts have very high nutritional value and increase digestive fire. This book makes use of sprouted mung beans.

Steam Sauté: To cook in a frying pan, covered, with a small amount of water and no oil.

Temper: To fry spices lightly in oil on medium heat, until they release essential oils, thereby increasing aroma and flavor and adding "temperance" to the dish. The spices and oil (called "tempering") are often poured into a dal or stew at the end of cooking.

Veggie Prep: To dice, slice, or coarsely chop vegetables and store in airtight glass containers for use the next day. Doing your veggie prep on a day off or a slow day is a great way to save time and still be able to cook fresh meals.

Seasonal Shopping Lists

Buy from the Everyday list year-round, and consult the at-a-glance seasonal lists for the extras you will want to stock for making the seasonal recipes.

EVERYDAY SHOPPING LIST

VEGETABLES
Beets
Carrots
Collards
Kale
Parsley, fresh
Swiss chard

FRUITS
Apples, in season
Lemons
Pears, in season

GRAINS
Brown basmati rice
White basmati rice

BEANS
Mung beans, green
Mung beans, split yellow

FATS
Butter, unsalted (to make ghee)

Chia seeds
Coconut oil
Flax oil
Flaxseeds
Hemp seeds
Olive oil
Sunflower seeds
Yogurt, fresh, whole milk

SPICES
Braggs Liquid Aminos
Cardamom powder
Cinnamon powder
Coriander seed
Cumin seed
Fennel seed
Ginger powder
Gingerroot
Pink salt

Sea salt
Tamari
Turmeric powder

EXTRAS
Ginger tea
Honey, raw (except in summer, see page 129)
Vegetable broth

SPRING SHOPPING LIST

VEGETABLES
Artichokes, fresh
Artichokes, marinated
Arugula
Asparagus
Cauliflower
Daikon radish
Endive
Leeks
Radicchio
Spinach
Sprouts

FRUITS
Apples
Berries, fresh
Cherries, dried
Cranberry juice
Grapefruit
Pears
Pomegranate juice
Prunes
Raisins

GRAINS
Amaranth
Barley
Buckwheat
Corn tortillas
Millet
Rye

BEANS
Black beans
Chickpeas
Green lentils
Red lentils

Tofu (firm)
White beans

FATS
Goat cheese
Rice milk
Soy milk

SPICES
Mustard seeds
Red chilies, dried
Sambar powder
Star anise

EXTRAS
Apple cider vinegar
Honey, raw
Rice vinegar

SUMMER SHOPPING LIST

VEGETABLES	FRUITS	GRAINS	FATS	SPICES
Beets	Apples	Barley	Avocados	Cardamom
Corn	Berries	Quinoa	Coconut,	Coriander
Cucumbers	Dates		shredded	Fennel
Fennel	Melons	BEANS	Coconut milk	Turmeric
Herbs (parsley,	Peaches	Chickpeas	Coconut oil	
cilantro, thyme,	Plums	White beans	Cow's cheese	EXTRAS
basil, mint, dill)			Goat cheese	Chickpea flour
Lettuce			Yogurt	Coconut water
Summer squash				Hemp protein
Zucchini				Rose water

FALL SHOPPING LIST

VEGETABLES		GRAINS	FATS	SPICES
Beets	Swiss chard	Brown rice	Avocados	Cardamom
Broccoli	Turnips	Oats (rolled	Coconut,	Cloves
Carrots		and steel cut)	shredded	
Collards	FRUITS	Red rice	Coconut milk	EXTRAS
Kale	Apples	Wheat	Cow's milk	Cacao powder
Parsnips	Bananas		Eggs	Coconut sugar
Pumpkins	Cranberries	BEANS	Goat's milk	Maple syrup
Spinach	Dates	Adzuki beans	Raw nut butters	
Squashes	Figs	Black beans	Raw nuts	
	Pears		Tahini	
	Raisins			

WINTER SHOPPING LIST

VEGETABLES			FATS	SPICES
Artichokes	Swiss chard	Pears	Almond meal	Chili powder
Beets	Tomatoes,		Cashews	Paprika
Carrots	farm-canned	GRAINS	Coconut,	Red chilies, dried
Collards	Yams	Brown rice	shredded	
Kale		Bulgur wheat	Cow's milk	EXTRAS
Parsnips	FRUITS	Oats	Eggs	Apple cider
Potatoes	Apples	Red rice	Goat's milk	vinegar
Roasted red	Bananas	Rice noodles	Sesame oil	Cacao powder
peppers	Dates		Sunflower butter	Maple syrup
Sea vegetables	Grapefruit	BEANS	Tahini	Molasses
Squashes	Mangoes	Black beans		Rice vinegar
Sweet potatoes	Oranges	Green lentils		
	Papayas	Red lentils		

Cooking Tables

Everyday Bean Cookery

The most efficient way to use beans is to plan ahead a day or two, cook up a good-sized batch (starting with 2 cups of dry beans), and make two different recipes with them. One cup of cooked beans can be used to make burgers, croquettes, a pâté recipe, or served atop an Everyday Steamed Salad Bowl (page 94). Beans served in their own broth over a grain make a great simple dish, and a chutney on the side adds some color.

CHOOSING HOME COOKED OVER CANNED

Canned foods of any kind have less vitality than fresh and so will sit more heavily in the body than ones you have cooked yourself. If you are in a pinch, however, it is better to prepare some food for yourself using the occasional canned goods than to eat out all the time. Please don't avoid beans because you think they take too much time to prepare. Simmering beans for a few hours is easy to do anytime that you happen to be around at home: in the morning, while you are preparing for the day; in the evening, relaxing after work or the evening meal; while you're doing laundry. And listen: if you aren't home for a few hours here and there during the week, consider that this is a sign of imbalance in itself.

MAKING A BATCH OF BEANS

Rinse all dry beans well before cooking.

In a fine mesh sieve, hold the beans under the water, moving the beans around with your fingers, until the water runs clear. (Kitchen hint: Talking to beans the way you talk to your plants makes cooking more fun.)

In a large pot, soak your beans for 8 to 12 hours in enough water to cover plus two inches. Watch for beans that float to the top or are discolored. These should be discarded. Add a chunk of kombu (about one inch of kombu for every cup of dry beans). This sea vegetable removes some of the gas from the beans, adds trace minerals, and makes a thick broth. (Forgot to soak? Check out the quick soak method on page 303.)

Cook your beans in the kombu water according to the chart timing, bringing to a boil uncovered first, then reducing heat to low, covering, and simmering. Check on your beans every half hour or so, adding hot

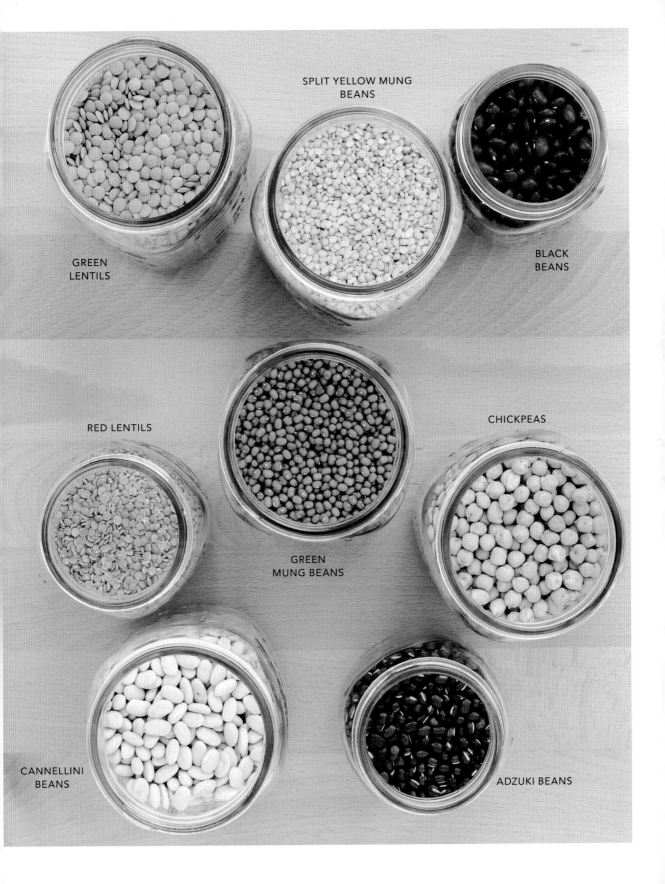

GREEN LENTILS

SPLIT YELLOW MUNG BEANS

BLACK BEANS

RED LENTILS

GREEN MUNG BEANS

CHICKPEAS

CANNELLINI BEANS

ADZUKI BEANS

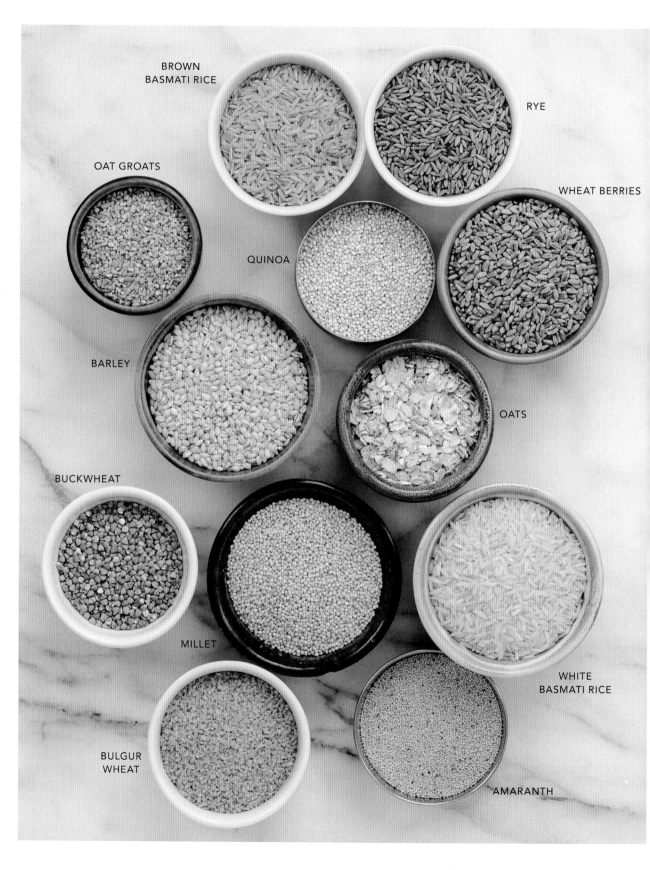

BROWN
BASMATI RICE

RYE

OAT GROATS

WHEAT BERRIES

QUINOA

BARLEY

OATS

BUCKWHEAT

MILLET

WHITE
BASMATI RICE

BULGUR
WHEAT

AMARANTH

water if needed to keep the beans covered. Cooking beans is not an exact science. Remember that once you are familiar with a type of bean, according to its seasonal effect and how you digest it, you will know through experience how soft it should be when cooked and about how long that takes. If you are prone to gassiness, stick to smaller beans and cook any bean until you can squish it completely between your fingers.

Cooking times will vary, depending on the age of the beans. Keep your stock fresh by rotating the contents of your bean pantry every season. Approximate cooking times are as follows.

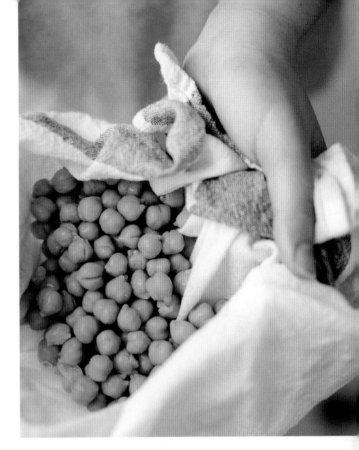

BEAN COOKING TIMES		
BEAN	COOKING TIME: SOAKED	COOKING TIME: DRY
Adzuki beans	45 minutes to 1 hour	60 to 90 minutes
Black beans	45 minutes to 1 hour	60 to 90 minutes
Cannellini beans	60 to 75 minutes	60 to 90 minutes
Chickpeas (garbanzos)	1½ to 2 hours	3+ hours
Red lentils	15 to 20 minutes	20 to 30 minutes
Split yellow mung beans	15 to 20 minutes	20 to 30 minutes
Whole mung beans	30 to 45 minutes	45 to 60 minutes

Cooking Grains

To cook grains, measure out your quantity of dry grain into a cooking pot and use the chart below to determine the amount of water or other liquid needed and the cooking time. Bring the liquid to a boil, then turn the heat down to low, cover tightly, and simmer until the liquid is absorbed.

GRAIN COOKING TIMES		
FOR EACH 1 CUP DRY	CUPS OF LIQUID	COOKING TIME
Barley (pearled)	2 ½	40 to 50 minutes
Brown rice	2	30 to 45 minutes
Buckwheat	2	15 minutes
Bulgur wheat	2	15 minutes
Millet	2	20 to 30 minutes
Oats, rolled	2	10 minutes
Oats, steel cut	3	30 minutes
Quinoa	1 ¾	15 to 20 minutes

As with beans, the cooking time can be reduced by presoaking grains for a few hours. Grains need not soak as long as beans, but you can soak them overnight. If you don't cook them within a day, refrigerate and cook within 2 days.

Measure the grain and water right into the pot you will cook in and let sit, covered. Cook time may reduce by as much as half, depending on the grain, so check your grain for tenderness early, if it is soaked.

NOTE: If you have a dry body type or it is fall/winter, it is beneficial to cook your grains with an extra ½ part water and to be in the habit of fluffing grains with a fork and ½ tsp of ghee or coconut oil per serving before enjoying.

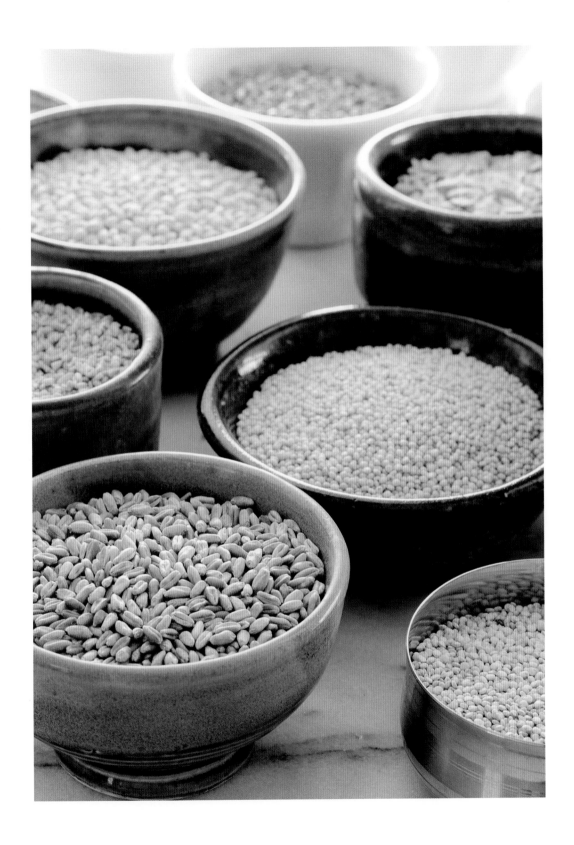

Recipe Index by Symptoms

Ayurveda works best when the diet and lifestyle change slowly over time—you can't just make a soup to instantly fix what is ailing you. But if you understand how the qualities of your meals can affect the way you feel, you're on the right track toward regaining health. This table offers a few recipe suggestions based on my own experience of using cooking as a home remedy.

SYMPTOM	QUALITIES THAT BALANCE	HELPFUL RECIPES
Acid indigestion	Cooling, dry, neutralizing, stable	Digestive Lassi, Fresh Fennel and Dill Soup, Everyday Kanjee, Cucumber Mint Raita, Cardamom Limeade
Anxiety	Warming, grounding, moist, soft, stable	Sweet Potato Bisque, Coconut Buttercup Soup, Spiced Nut Milk Smoothie, Winter Rejuvenating Tonic, Sunbutter Truffles
Congestion	Warming, dry, light, sharp, penetrating, mobile	South Indian Sambar, Refresh-O-Rama, Cleansing Green Juice, Spicy Andhra-Style Dal, Barley Kanjee, Spring Digestive Tea
Constipation	Warming, grounding, moist, oily	Everyday Chia Pudding, Everyday Cleansing Green Soup, Stewed Apples with Dates, Ghee Fried Apples, Raw Beet Slaw with Lemon and Mint

SYMPTOM	QUALITIES THAT BALANCE	HELPFUL RECIPES
Dry skin	Warming, grounding, moist, oily	Ghee, Chocolate Bark, Everyday Almond Milk, Everyday Chia Pudding
Gas and bloating	Warming, grounding, moist, soft	Everyday Kichari, Digestive Lassi, Fall Digestive Tea
Headaches	Cooling, dry, neutralizing, soft, slow	Everyday Kanjee, Everyday Kichari, Basil Melon Cooler, Detox Dal Soup
Lethargy, feeling unmotivated	Warming, light, sharp, mobile	Masala Chai, Cleansing Green Juice, Berry Buck-Up Cereal
Red skin, inflammation	Cooling, dry, neutralizing, stable	Cleansing Green Juice, Everyday Cleansing Green Soup, Detox Dal Soup, The Beet Queen, Cilantro Mint Chutney
Sleeping difficulty	Warming, grounding, moist, soft, stable	Winter Rejuvenating Tonic, Everyday Kichari, Spiced Nut Milk Smoothie
Water retention, puffiness	Light, dry, sharp, penetrating, mobile	Barley Kanjee, Cherry Millet Cakes, Easy Chana Dosa, Detox Dal Soup, Cranberry Clove Chutney

Notes

CHAPTER 1

1. Vagbhata, Ashtanga Hridayam, Sutrasthana 1.6. "The dosha are material substances in the body always, they have their own definite quantity, quality, and functions. When they are normal they attend to different functions of the body and so maintain it. But they have the tendency to become abnormal undergoing increase or decrease in their quantity, one or more of their qualities and functions ... because of this tendency to vitiation [disorder], they are called as doshas."
2. Vagbhata, Ashtanga Hridayam, vol. 1, Sutrasthana 12.34-42.
3. Agniveśa, Charaka Samhita, vol. 1, Sutrasthana 30.8. Trans. Dr. Ram Karan Sharma and Vaidya Bhagwan Dash (Varanasi: Chowkhamba Krishnadas Academy).
4. AKA Charita Samhita, Sutrasthana 30.9.

CHAPTER 2

1. Vagbhata, Ashtanga Hridayam, vol. 1, Sutrasthana 8.49. Trans. Prof. K. R. Srikantha Murthy, 6th ed. (Varanasi: Chowkhamba Krishnadas Academy, 2009).

CHAPTER 8

1. Vagbhata, Ashtanga Hridayam, vol. 1, Sutrasthana 2.8-9. Trans. Prof. K. R. Srikantha Murthy, 6th ed. (Varanasi: Chowkhamba Krishnadas Academy, 2009).

Glossary

Sanskrit Terms

Abhyanga: A massage in which one applies warm oil to the body using strokes in a specific pattern to support movements of energy according to Ayurvedic principles.

Agni: The fire element; also refers to the digestive fire.

Ahara Rasa: The nutritive liquid resulting from chewing and digesting food; the building block of all bodily tissue.

Ama: A thick, sticky by-product of incomplete digestion; in Ayurveda it is believed to be the root of all disease.

Amla: Sour taste; combination of fire and earth elements.

Charaka Samhita: The principal texts of Ayurveda, said to be three thousand years old, and still the main reference sources for most Ayurvedic practitioners.

Dal: A classic soupy Indian dish made from any variety of legumes. Originally the term referred to the legume of the pigeon pea bush, known as *tur dal*.

Deepana: To kindle digestive fire.

Dinacharya: Literally, "to follow the day"; used to reference daily routines that establish balance.

Dosha: That which causes imbalance; essential biological compounds present in the body.

Gunas: Qualities or attributes found in the five elements and therefore in all things.

Kapha: The energy of structure and lubrication, cohesion; combination of earth and water elements.

Kashaya: Astringent taste; combination of air and earth elements.

Katu: Pungent taste; combination of fire and air elements.

Kichari: A general term in Ayurveda for a soupy rice and legume dish.

Lavana: Salty taste; combination of fire and water elements.

Madhura: Sweet taste; combination of water and earth elements.

Nasya: To administer medicines through the nasal cavity.

Neti: To irrigate the nasal passage with saline water, usually using a special vessel called a neti pot.

Ojas: Literally, "vigor"; the cream of the nutrient fluid in the body; the essence of immunity.

Pachana: To digest; in Ayurveda, a means to improve digestion.

Panchakarma: Literally, "five actions"; an Ayurvedic detoxification treatment using five different methods.

Pancha Mahabhutas: The five great elements; ether, air, fire, water, earth.

Pitta: That which transforms or digests; combination of fire and water elements.

Prajnaparadha: Crimes against wisdom.

Prana: Vital energy of the universe.

Rasayana: Literally, "path of essence"; the science of lengthening the life span; a medicinal combination of substances to improve immunity.

Rtucharya: Seasonal regimen; the changing of the seasons.

Sattva: The energy of peace, clarity, and inspiration.

Tejas: Metabolic energy; the subtle energetic essence of pitta; gives luster to the body.

Thali: A meal consisting of rice and several regional meat or vegetable dishes.

Tikta: Bitter; combination of ether and air elements.

Vata: That which moves; combination of air and ether elements.

Vipak: The postdigestive effect a substance has on the body.

Uncommon Ingredients

Almond Meal: Raw almonds, skin and all, ground into a powder to be used as a flour; high in protein; also called almond flour.

Apple Cider Vinegar: A higher acid vinegar made from fermented apples. Unfiltered, it retains more nutrients.

Asafetida: A traditional Ayurvedic spice, strong tasting, used in place of onion and garlic; also known as hing.

Ashwagandha: A deeply revitalizing tonic in Ayurveda; the root is powdered and dried for medicinal use; commonly known as Indian ginseng and Indian winter cherry.

Bragg Liquid Aminos: A nonfermented soybean sauce.

Cacao Powder: The cacao bean is shelled, dried and fermented, and broken into bits called nibs, which are cold pressed and ground to make cacao powder. This process maintains nutrition that is otherwise destroyed when the cacao is roasted to make cocoa powder.

Cardamom Pods: A cooling spice often used in sweets and beverages; available in black and green pods. This book calls for the seeds found inside the green pods.

Chickpea Flour: Dried chickpeas ground into flour; high in protein; a common ingredient in Indian sweets. Can be found at Indian markets and in bulk at natural foods stores.

Coconut Flour: The fiber, protein, and fat remaining in the coconut meat after oil extraction, which is ground to a powder that can be used as a flour.

Coconut Sugar Crystals: A sugar produced by tapping the flowers of the coconut palm to withdraw the nectar; available in block, syrup, and granular forms.

Coconut Water: The sweet, cooling water from the inside of the young green coconut; whole coconuts are cracked open so the water can be drunk through a straw. Packaged coconut water is now available in stores for a treat.

Cold-Pressed Coconut Oil: Oil that has been removed from the meat of the fresh coconut through cold pressing. This method does not introduce heat, which can make the oil rancid.

Dulse: A salty sea vegetable that grows on cold coasts, such as those of the United States, Japan, and England. Dulse is red in color when dried; very high in B vitamins.

Gingerroot: The rhizome of the ginger plant; can be used fresh, as well as in dried and powdered forms.

Green Mung Beans: Small, green-skinned beans prized in Ayurveda for their ability to nourish the body without encouraging any imbalances.

Kabocha Squash: A sweet Asian variety of winter squash with thin green skin and orange flesh; related to the Hubbard and Buttercup varieties. The term can also refer to other varieties of Asian winter squashes.

Kombu: An edible kelp harvested on ropes in the oceans of Japan and Korea.

Legume: A type of plant that grows edible seeds inside pods; commonly called beans or pulses.

Medjool Date: A variety of date from hot, dry climates that retains some of its moisture after being packaged; more moist and sweet than the deglet noor variety.

Miso: A salty, fermented paste made from legumes and grains, commonly soybeans, barley, and chickpeas; widely used in Japanese cooking.

Mustard Seed Oil: An oil made from pressed mustard seeds; used in Ayurvedic massage to warm and mobilize conditions of heaviness or stagnation.

Nori: A sweet, dark green, highly nutritious sea vegetable, usually pressed into sheets for sushi.

Raw Honey: Honey that has not been cooked in processing. If a label does not state that it is raw, the product has been heated. Ayurveda considers cooked honey indigestible and a potential toxin.

Rice Vinegar: A Chinese, Japanese, Korean, and Vietnamese condiment made from fermented rice; milder and sweeter than most Western vinegars.

Saffron: An orange-colored spice commonly used in Indian sweets; in cooking the stamens of the plants, called threads, are used. Saffron is a blood purifier.

Sambar Powder: Red in color, a coarse, powdered combination of roasted lentils, dried whole red chilies, fenugreek seeds, coriander seeds, asafetida, curry leaves, cumin, black pepper, and other spices; used in tomato-based soups.

Sesame Oil: The oil cold pressed from sesame seeds. Can be purchased in toasted, raw, and refined forms; for massage buy organic oil that is refined for medium heat.

Split Mung Beans: Green mung beans with their skin removed, split in half; light yellow in color.

Tahini: A paste made by grinding sesame seeds; can be found made of roasted or raw seeds.

Tamari: A salty, fermented soybean condiment, very much like soy sauce, but wheat free.

Tamarind: A tree native to Africa, now cultivated in other tropical regions. A paste can be made from its partially dried fruits. Extremely sour, the fruit has both culinary and medicinal uses.

Tonic: A medicinal substance taken to increase a feeling of vigor and well-being.

Tulsi: A medicinal plant of Indian origin, commonly used to boost the immune and respiratory systems; also known as holy basil; widely available as a tea.

Ume Plum Vinegar: A Japanese condiment, the brine by-product of the pickling of umeboshi plums; contains salt and red *shiso* leaf. Tastes are salty, sour, and sweet.

Unrefined, Dehydrated, Whole Cane Sugar: A sugar produced by pressing the juice from sugarcane and dehydrating it to make brown crystals. This product is more nutritious than conventional white or brown sugar. It has different names in different parts of the world. In Ayurveda, it is called jaggery; also known as Sucanat (a brand name), rapadura, muscovado.

Resources for Ingredients, Experiences, and Education

Favorite Suppliers of Spices, Sea Vegetables, and Ghee

Maine Coast Sea Vegetables
Sustainably harvested seaweeds from the North Atlantic
www.seaveg.com

Mountain Rose Herbs
Organic herbs and spices
www.mountainroseherbs.com

Pure Indian Foods
Certified organic grassfed ghee and organic spices
www.pureindianfoods.com

Ayurvedic Suppliers for Dinacharya

For special discount codes visit ayurvedicliving.institute/our-favorites or follow Kate O'Donnell on social media.

The Ayurvedic Institute
Ayurvedic herbs and spices, massage oils, nasya oil
store.ayurveda.com

Banyan Botanicals
Ayurvedic herbs and spices, massage oils, nasya oil, neti pot
www.banyanbotanicals.com

Farmtrue
Small-batch organic ghee, massage oils, spices, natural bath and body, and dinacharya kits
www.farmtrue.com

Organic Produce

Environmental Working Group
"Dirty Dozen" and "Clean Fifteen" annual guides to pesticides in produce
www.ewg.org

USDA National Farmers Market Directory
www.nfmd.org

Experiences: Ayurveda Clinics and Retreat Centers

These are resources I have direct experience with, and there are so many others. Research in your local area may uncover a gem. Please tell them we sent you!

PANCHAKARMA IN INDIA
Sitaram Beach Retreat
sitaramretreat.com

Vaidyagrama Healing Center
www.vaidyagrama.com

PANCHAKARMA IN THE UNITED STATES
North Carolina
The Ayurvedic Institute
www.ayurveda.com

Vermont
The Ayurvedic Center of Vermont
www.ayurvedavermont.com

Find an Ayurvedic Practitioner

United States

National Ayurvedic Medical Association

http://ayurvedanama.org

UK

Ayurvedic Professionals Association - UK

https://apa.uk.com/find-a-member

Europe

Association of European Ayurvedic Doctors and Therapists

www.ayurveda-verband.eu/en/aerztetherapeuten/search-doctorstherapists/

Ayurveda Education and Training

Ayurvedic Living Institute

ayurvedicliving.institute

The Ayurvedic Institute

www.ayurveda.com

California College of Ayurveda

www.ayurvedacollege.com

Kripalu School of Ayurveda

www.kripalu.org

Acknowledgments

I would like to thank many people for supporting *The Everyday Ayurveda Cookbook* from start to finish. First of all is Cara Brostrom, whose contributions go far beyond photography alone. She and I would like to thank all those who rallied around us through this process. A hearty thank you and thumbs-up to:

The folks at Shambhala Publications and, most of all, the book midwife Rochelle Bourgault.

The Ayurvedic readers and editors: Dr. Robert Svoboda, Hilary Garivaltis, Erin Casperson (triple gold star), Kristen Rae Stevens, and Bobbie Jo Allen.

Two special contributors who celebrated in the kitchen with Cara and me and suffered incompatible food combinations in the name of Ayurveda: Erin Casperson and Risa Horn.

Our designer, Allison Meierding, who has been behind this book from its inception.

Suppliers of fine linens: Wendi Wing, Dorothy Fennell, and Allison Meierding.

Suppliers of Ayurvedic products: Pure Indian Foods and Banyan Botanicals.

The testers: Risa Horn, Dane Smith, Allison Meierding, Erin Casperson, Patty Crotty, Lauren Varney, Bristol Maryott, Bharti Thakkar, Emily Griffin, Beth Rausch, Birgit Wurster, Ellise Basch, Rich Ray.

The sharp eye of Laura Shaw Feit.

The nannies: Emily Morris and Shannon Maguire. And to Beth Brostrom for traveling to Boston to look after the baby as deadlines approached.

The family: Mom and Dad O'Donnell for telling me how fantastic the book was from day one. To Rich Ray and Chris and Evelyn Okerberg for their unconditional love and support.

To my yoga and Ayurveda gurus and to all the yoga students and Ayurvedic clients for their support along the way.

Index

About Us

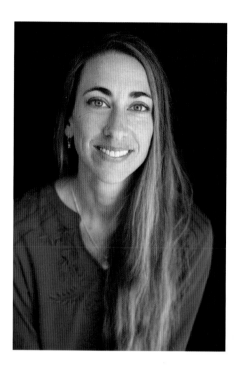

Kate O'Donnell has spent more than twenty-five years traveling through India in search of ancient, time-tested, healing practices to bring back to the United States. Through her own healing journey, Kate experienced firsthand how a holistic system creates lasting health. She's since emerged as a preeminent expert in Ayurveda—the sister science to yoga—and has built her own curriculum customized for modern Americans. Her individualized approach—"guiding from disease to ease"—has transformed the lives of thousands of people and made her a respected thought leader in holistic medicine. Kate's best-selling books, published in seven languages, continue to be top resources in the field of Ayurveda. As a highly sought-after speaker and the founder of the Ayurvedic Living Institute, she has educated a generation of practitioners.

Thousands continue to heal with Kate through her annual detox programs, community education, and retreats and are inspired to radiant health by her teachings as well as her example. Find Kate at https://ayurvedicliving.institute, and follow her on Instagram @kateodonnell.ayurveda for daily inspiration.

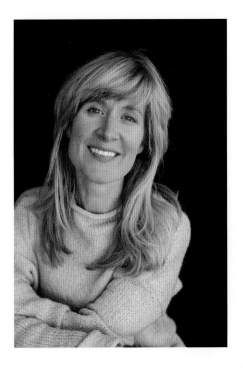

Cara Brostrom is an artist, writer, and photographer. Her work has been exhibited throughout Europe and North America and published in magazines, newspapers, blogs, and websites online and in print. Over ten years ago, during many early mornings at a yoga studio in Boston with Kate O'Donnell, *The Everyday Ayurveda Cookbook* was cooked up as an idea and brought to life in Kate and Cara's small apartment kitchens, one recipe and one photograph at a time. In the years that followed, Cara has continued to study and practice Ayurveda, yoga, and bioregional herbalism and photographed and consulted on *Everyday Ayurveda Cooking for a Calm, Clear Mind*, *The Everyday Ayurveda Guide to Self-Care*, and *Everyday Ayurveda for Women's Health*. Cara lives with her family in Western Massachusetts. Learn more at www.carabrostrom.com.

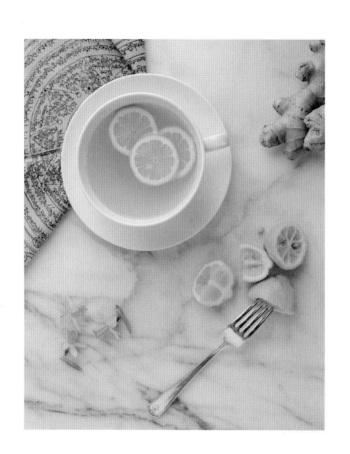